A business approach to facilities

NATIONAL HEALTH SERVICE IN SCOTLAND ESTATES ENVIRONMENT FORUM

NHS Estates
An Executive Agency of the Department of Health

First published 1998

ISBN 0-11-322151-7

Standing order service

Are you making full use of The Stationery Office's Standing Order Service?

The Standing Order Service is a free monitoring of the publications of your choice from over 4000 classifications in 30 major subject areas. We send you your books as they are published, along with an invoice.

With a standing order for class 14.02.024 you can be supplied automatically with further titles in this series as they are published.

The benefits to you are:

- automatic supply of your choice of classification on publication;
- no need for time-consuming and costly research, telephone calls and scanning of daily publication lists;
- saving on the need and the costs of placing individual orders.

We can supply a wide range of publications on standing order, from individual annual publications to all publications on a selected subject. If you do not already use this free service, or think you are not using it to its full capacity, why not contact us and discuss your requirements?

You can contact us at:

The Stationery Office
Standing Order Department
PO Box 276
London SW8 5DT

Tel: 0171-873 8466; fax 0171-873 8222

We look forward to hearing from you.

About this series

Health Facilities Notes (HFNs) address topical subjects, often in response to NHS-driven initiatives, and aim to provide an insight into issues. They may draw widely from, and challenge, trends in the UK, Europe and North America. HFNs do not include formal policy input from the Department of Health.

In many cases, HFNs consider a wide range of alternative options and the implications of those options in terms of cost consequence and acceptability to users.

Executive summary

This HFN provides guidance on developing a business approach to facilities management (FM). By tracing the development of FM in five very different trusts around the UK, this document identifies the key features of a successful FM service.

FM is defined as 'the process by which an NHS trust creates and sustains a caring environment and delivers quality hotel services to meet clinical needs at best cost'. Although FM services may be provided in a variety of ways – ranging from in-house delivery and management to completely outsourced FM services – the principles upon which the FM process is based are broadly similar. Evidence suggests that the most successful FM services are those that are planned and developed across the whole organisation. In other words, FM must be supported at all levels: corporate, strategic, tactical and operational.

Corporate. The opportunities for developing FM will be determined by the corporate culture and management structure. Traditional, hierarchical cultures cannot be changed into service-oriented cultures overnight but it is possible, as a first step, to consider how the existing culture may be exploited or to what extent organisational barriers can be removed. The trust's senior management team determines the healthcare objectives and sets the business targets; it is at this level that the conditions for successful FM are set. It is important that FM managers are able to influence these strategic decisions.

Strategic. The actions required at this level relate to business planning, the development of an FM policy, and the appointment of an "intelligent client" to promote and represent the FM function internally and externally. The FM strategy should be supported by a marketing plan, customer feedback mechanisms, and a well designed and accurate information system.

Tactical. Programmes to manage quality, value and risk must be introduced.

Quality – A range of measures is required, including total quality management programmes, self-assessment, team working, multi-skilling and staff empowerment.

Value – Assessing the value of a service requires accurate methods of measuring performance, for example benchmarking.

Risk – FM managers may be well placed to take the lead in developing a risk management strategy for the trust as a whole.

Operational. FM services must be monitored to ensure that the day-to-day business is kept on track. This is done by setting a number of key indicators against which performance can be assessed.

This four level approach is used as a framework for analysing the development of FM in each of the selected case studies. The document concludes that there are four key requirements for successful FM:

- effective corporate management;
- the appointment of an intelligent client;
- continual process improvement;
- organisational development.

Bringing all these elements together to create an environment in which FM can flourish is a difficult task which may take many months or even years. However, the reward is continually improving services and satisfied patients.

Acknowledgements

NHS Estates would like to thank the following people for their contribution to this document:

Keith Alexander, director, Centre for Facilities Management, University of Strathclyde, Glasgow;

Mike Gallagher, director of facilities, Blackpool Victoria Hospital NHS Trust, Lancashire;

Stephen Harrup, director of estates and facilities, Ipswich Hospital NHS Trust, Suffolk;

Colin G Hillyard, formerly director of estates, Southern Derbyshire Health Authority, Secretary, Health Estates and Facilities Managers Association;

Phil Rickett, Worcestershire Community Healthcare NHS Trust;

Louise McGrath, research fellow, Centre for Facilities Management, University of Strathclyde, Glasgow;

David Browning, director of facilities, Hairmyres & Stonehouse NHS Trust, East Kilbride, Lanarkshire;

Geoff Callan, Milton Keynes General NHS Trust, Buckinghamshire;

Jennifer Cowpe, Worcestershire Community Healthcare NHS Trust;

Janet Marriot, Worcestershire Community Healthcare NHS Trust;

Jim Hawley, Northampton Community Healthcare Trust;

Chris Simms, Blackpool Victoria Hospital NHS Trust, Lancashire.

Contents

1.0 Introduction

Purpose of this document

This Health Facilities Note (HFN) provides guidance on developing a business approach to Facilities Management (FM). It builds upon HFN 16 – 'Re-engineering the facilities management service' by describing in detail the processes and actions required at all organisational levels – from corporate to operational – to ensure a successful and professional FM service. The document illustrates how these processes can be applied and draws conclusions about best practice by examining very different examples of FM in five NHS trusts.

A self-assessment checklist is provided as a practical tool enabling trusts to assess FM performance in their own organisation.

Facilities management in context

Facilities management in the NHS is relatively mature. Over the past decade it has grown and developed in response to the NHS reforms and the creation of the internal market. The publication of the White Paper 'A new NHS', however, provides a new context for the development of FM: the emphasis has shifted away from competition towards partnership and collaboration. The White Paper highlights the need for quality and efficiency across the whole NHS:

> 'Every part of the NHS, and everyone who works in it, should take responsibility for working to improve quality. This must be quality in its broadest sense: doing the right things at the right time, for the right people, and doing them right – first time. And it must be the quality of the patient's experience as well as the clinical result – quality measured in terms of prompt access, good relationships and efficient administration.'

This philosophy recognises that a patient's perception of quality is based not only on clinical treatments but also on a range of other factors relating to the overall healthcare experience. Support functions, such as catering, cleaning, administration and reception services, can create lasting first impressions – good and bad. Improving the quality of these services is an integral part of improving healthcare services in general.

The NHS has seen a gradual evolution from ad hoc engineering and works operations to planned and developmental estates management and finally towards a strategic approach to all non-clinical services. Today FM is primarily about responding to patients' needs.

A 1993 survey of FM practice in the NHS revealed that most FM departments adopted a site-oriented approach, with managers having responsibility for a greater number of buildings than their counterparts in the private sector. Responsibilities for support services covered a wider range than in other sectors because of the definition of non-clinical activities in the NHS. The results of a similar survey in 1995 are summarised in Table 1.

Facilities plan	40% of trusts surveyed have a written facilities plan with an average planning period of 1-3 years
Responsibilities	Typically include building management, telecoms, property management and environmental management
Average budget	£8.8 million
Service level agreements	Used in 74% of trusts surveyed, with 56% being initiated by facilities managers
Contracting out	A major trend with 45% of trusts surveyed indicating an increase in activity
Contract durations	Short to medium-term contracts (1 to 3 years) are most common (63% of trusts surveyed)
Partnering	Not seen as a general trend, with only 16% of trusts surveyed using partnerships
Tender evaluation criteria	Cost/price and quality are the most commonly used criteria

Table 1: Survey of FM practice in the NHS, 1995

Source: Study of facilities management practice in the UK 1994/95, Part 1: Facilities management practice in the NHS (1995). Centre for Facilities Management, not published

Definition of facilities management

HFN 16 suggests that the purpose of FM is to increase the value of services, either by improving the quality of service for the same cost, or delivering the same service for a lower cost – or a combination of both. In order to achieve this, facilities managers must have an understanding of the broad context in which services are operated. They should consider the range and scope of services offered, the markets for those services, and the structure of the organisation. This document extends this thinking, and emphasises the need to consider the ways in which facilities contribute to healthcare and to effective business.

The working definition of FM adopted in HFN 16 is that proposed by the US Library of Congress:

> 'the practice of co-ordinating the physical workplace with the people and work of the organisation; (it) integrates the principles of business administration, architecture, and the behavioural and engineering sciences'.

This definition highlights three key facets of FM:

- it is a supporting function to the core business of the organisation;
- it focuses on the interface between the physical workplace and people; and
- it requires a multi-skill approach.

HFN 16 concludes that successful facilities must be strategically planned and a clear relationship shown between the development of FM and the operational and business needs of the trust as a whole. This HFN develops the themes further by focusing on strategic issues and upon processes that ensure facilities support healthcare objectives. For the purposes of this document, therefore, FM in the NHS may be defined as

> 'the process by which an NHS trust creates and sustains a caring environment and delivers quality hotel services to meet clinical needs at best cost'.

Models of facilities management

In 'Contracting for competitive NHS support services' four models of FM are identified:

- A traditional approach where the majority of services are delivered and managed in-house. A small number of specialist contracts may be controlled and integrated by the FM manager.
- A balanced approach between in-house services and out-sourced functions, plus specialist contracts. In this model, entire services such as catering or maintenance may be contracted out, while others are retained in-house.
- An entirely out-sourced FM package using either one major contractor or a limited number of smaller contractors. An in-house FM manager is responsible for overseeing the operation.
- A PFI model where the complete FM package is out-sourced through a management contract with an external facilities manager acting on the trust's behalf.

Figure 1 illustrates the options available to trusts wishing to use external FM suppliers.

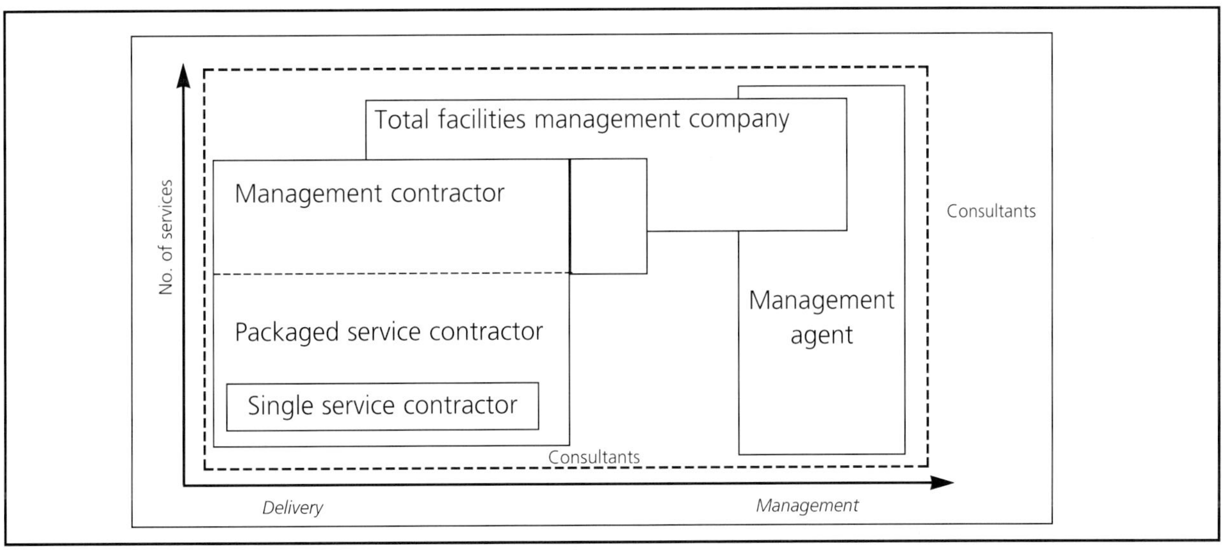

Figure 1: Framework of the facilities management industry
Source: Facilities management industry analysis: Issue 2 (1996). Centre for Facilities Management, not published

Notes:

Single service contracting – companies concentrate on the delivery of one particular service type.

Packaged service contracting – companies draw together a variety of types of service to provide a range of service delivery.

Management contracting – companies provide a balance of delivery and management and tend to focus on a small number of service types. Client organisations tend to deal with a number of management contractors and retain overall management control.

Total Facilities Management (TFM) – companies may deliver and manage a wide range of services either directly or by sub-contract. They offer clients a comprehensive service and their emphasis is on management ability. In such cases the client relinquishes the hands-on management of facilities.

Management agency – agents provide a "management only" service. Where a management agent is appointed by a client, they will tend to contract directly with those companies delivering facilities.

Consultants – companies offer advice across a range of services, generally project related. Often involved at the "front-end" of the out-sourcing process, consultants tend to be brought in during transitional periods.

2.0 The facilities management process

Introduction

Although models of FM vary considerably, the principles upon which the process is based are generally very similar. For FM to be successful it must be considered at four levels:

At a **corporate level**, senior managers with responsibility for facilities must contribute to service planning, formulate policy and undertake scenario planning. This requires a full understanding of the corporate culture and responsibilities.

At a **strategic level**, managers carry responsibility for effective business planning of the facilities services, leadership of the team and the development of proposals for developing facilities.

At a **tactical level**, the facilities manager ensures service quality, manages value and implements risk management strategies.

At an **operational level**, the facilities manager ensures control through auditing and monitoring performance. Responsibilities for delivering an innovative service should be effectively delegated to service providers.

This Chapter describes in more detail the activities at each level, while Chapter 4 goes on to examine the FM process in five case studies.

A. Corporate level

Corporate culture

Corporate culture describes the values and beliefs of an organisation and its employees. Behavioural norms will be shaped by the social and political/economic environment in which the organisation operates, as well as by society's expectations.

FM has to operate within the corporate culture. Customary ways of gaining compliance, allowing discretion, evaluating performance and motivating staff are all important to a facilities manager who is attempting to alter people's attitudes and behaviour.

There are four distinct organisational cultures, as illustrated in Figure 2.

The cultural climate of an organisation will change according to environmental uncertainty and the time-scales in which it needs to operate.

Most healthcare organisations are fundamentally hierarchical cultures with strong, ordered structures and employees who are motivated by predictability and security. Such organisations are inward-looking and planning is long-term. Leadership is conservative with authority governed by rules and accountability formalised by systems of representation. In making decisions people tend to take a long time to gather and analyse information to reach the single optimal solution.

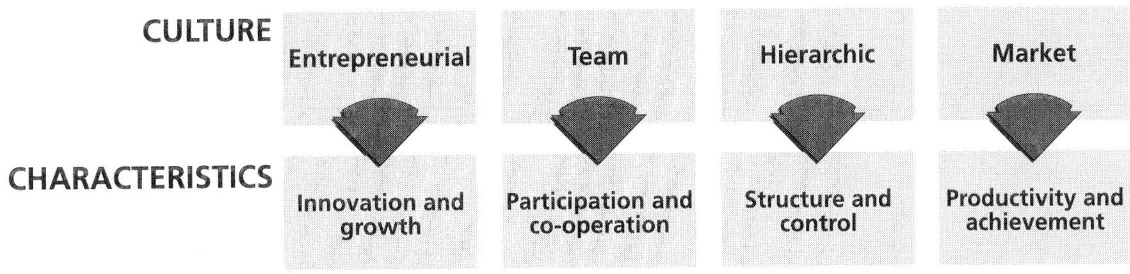

Figure 2: Organisational cultures and their characteristics

With the advent of trust status and under the influence of the NHS reforms, trusts are being driven to become more market-oriented. However, bringing about such cultural change requires the support of both employees and stakeholders and will take time to achieve.

Individuals are not equally comfortable in each of these cultural climates. A person with a need for achievement will prefer a market culture which demands immediate action and where certainty is high. A person with a need for affiliation will probably prefer a team culture where there is less need for action and less certainty and the emphasis is on co-operation. Particular managerial styles will suit particular cultures and this has important implications for facilities managers.

Identifying the corporate culture can help facilities manager to decide the most appropriate strategy and style to adopt in motivating people and altering their attitudes and behaviour. The kinds of question facilities managers need to ask are:

- to what extent can you exploit the existing culture of the organisation?
- are there ways round organisational constraints that impede progress?
- can you or should you attempt to change the organisation?
- to what extent should you accommodate the organisation?

Corporate management structure

The chief executive, board members and senior managers in the trust create the organisational climate within which all the healthcare and supporting activities are carried out. They determine healthcare objectives and set the "business" targets, within the legal bounds of the trust and the available resources. They decide on the size, shape and structure of the organisation needed to deliver the service.

It is at this level that the conditions for effective FM are set. It is important for facilities managers to have an influence on these strategic decisions and to demonstrate the contribution that facilities make to achieving the healthcare objectives and business targets.

The need for senior management support is clear. A recent study (Rees, 1997) assessed the extent to which the directors of FM are in a position to influence the trust's strategic development, business planning and policy decision-making. The seniority of directors of FM within their trusts was also evaluated. The study concluded that most directors of FM are members of the trust management team and can make a direct contribution to the development of their trust's strategy and its major policy decisions.

Figure 3 illustrates a typical organisational structure of an NHS trust. It is essential that there are clear lines of reporting and accountability and that the delegation of responsibility is unambiguous. The chief executive is ultimately accountable for many aspects of FM, including health and safety and other key risks. However, the facilities manager will carry nominated responsibility for specific aspects, such as fire safety.

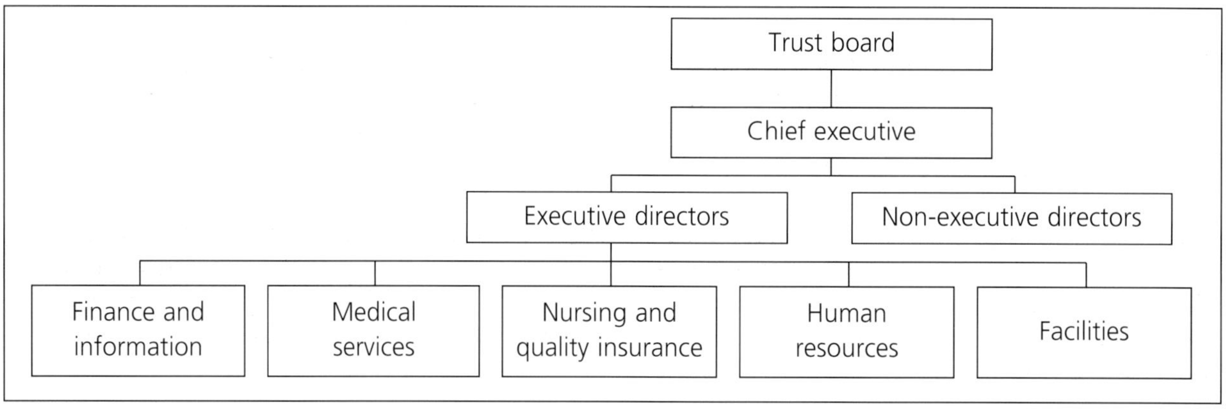

Figure 3: Typical organisational structure of an NHS trust

The key to successful FM, however, is not the technical ability of the facilities manager, but his or her management skills. Without managerial training and expertise, it will be difficult to raise the profile of FM within the trust.

B. Strategic level

Strategic planning

Strategic planning encompasses the trust's business direction, infrastructure and business environment. A strategic plan is long term, typically three to five years, and sets the context for the organisation's annual plans.

The FM strategic plan is usually articulated through a mission statement, which focuses on the role of FM in meeting the trust's overall business objectives.

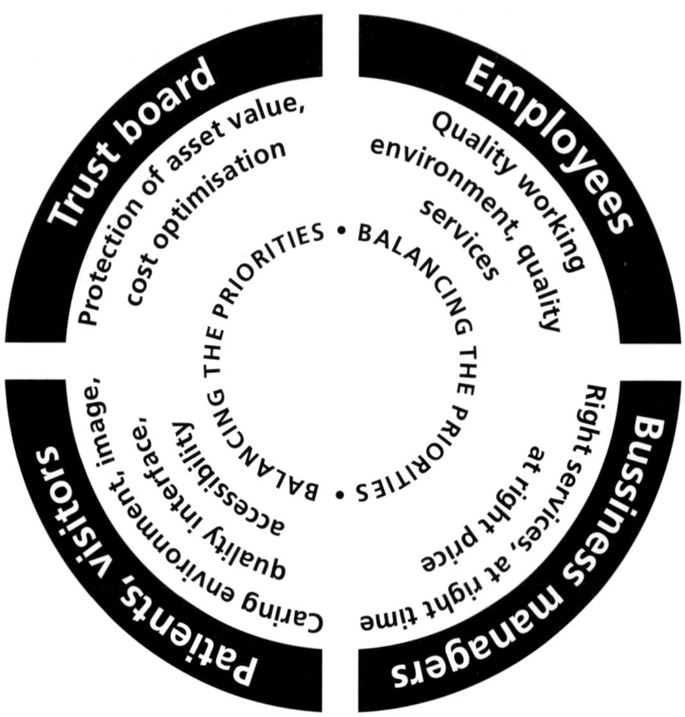

Figure 4: Balancing the priorities

The main aim of many FM departments is to provide customers with high quality and cost-effective services. Analysing customer requirements and perceptions is an important element in developing a strategic plan, and can be achieved through interviews, surveys, or customer feedback mechanisms such as complaint logs and help desks. While the overall customer is the trust, however, there are distinct groups of clients with different priorities, as shown in Figure 4.

The distillation of these various inputs creates the context, or situation statement, for the current year's plans. If the organisation is to be focused in a common direction, both situation statement and strategic objectives should be directly linked to those of the business units. For each key strategy, an implementation plan is developed which details the steps to be taken, the timescales and owners of each element. This allows for easy tracking during the course of the year.

The intelligent client

An "intelligent client" is a person employed by the trust to act as a single point of contact for clients and to represent their interests. The role of the intelligent client will normally include:

- formulating policy;
- gaining influence in the organisation;
- contributing to the strategic decision making process;
- creating a service culture;
- raising the profile (marketing);
- building relationships with stakeholders;
- designing systems and frameworks;
- securing funding.

The intelligent client should understand the business of FM – not just its operation, but also its values and long-term goals. He/she co-ordinates views within the organisation and, if necessary, interprets the market for external service providers. The intelligent client should command strong organisational support and should occupy a senior executive position, with a voice in the boardroom.

Developing an FM policy

Many trusts, even those well advanced in FM, have not as yet found it necessary to have a formal policy for FM. Without a written policy, however, the trust's attempts to manage facilities will be vulnerable to changes in personnel and/or alterations in perceived priorities.

The purpose of the facilities policy is to set out the mission, remit and objectives of FM. It will lay down FM/business performance indicators, roles and responsibilities, decision-making and reporting structure, and communication procedures.

Part 1

Declaration of top management commitment to, and senior and middle management's involvement in FM;

Statement of policy;

Statement of objectives, separated into short- and long-term goals.

Part 2

An action plan, specifying a time-tabled programme of work;

Costed resource requirements, including staff complement, investment and training needs, necessary to achieve the programme;

Assigned responsibility and accountability for actions outlined, specifying individuals by name and post;

Description of FM committee's remit, structure, membership and reporting mechanisms;

Named committee representative for each department and specification of internal and external lines of communication;

Statement of review procedure, defining milestones and mechanisms for assessing overall progress and value for money, as well as appraising the performance of individual members of staff.

Source: Centre for Facilities Management, unpublished

The facilities policy document can be organised in two parts – a policy declaration and an operating policy. The policy declaration is for publication and dissemination; while the detailed operating policy may contain commercially-sensitive information and is for internal circulation only. The operating policy is a working document to guide FM practices and provide continuity.

While it is the responsibility of the facilities manager to formulate the FM policy, it is likely to be more widely accepted if all relevant parties contribute to its formulation. The way the policy is drafted will depend not only on the trust's culture, but also on the facilities manager's own managerial style.

Once the policy has been formulated it is important that it be formally adopted and ratified within the organisation. Without this it may be difficult to access the resources required to support the FM activities.

Business planning

Planning is key to the success of any business. Without it, an organisation is trapped in reactive mode with little concern over its long-term future.

In the context of the strategic plan, financial plans/budgets and the previous year's performance are reviewed to define the current year's plan of action. The output of this stage is the annual breakthrough plan, which summarises the current situation, identifies objectives to address that situation and key strategies that will ensure success.

A typical business plan should include :

- executive summary;
- background;
- main services;
- market analysis;

- operations;
- management;
- organisation and personnel;
- ownership;
- financial analysis;
- risks and rewards;
- objectives and milestones;
- appendices.

Source: HFN 16: 'Re-engineering the facilities management service'. NHS Estates, SO 1996

Facilities managers work with three groups of customers – patients, employees and the team of facilities service providers. Typically when translating plans into action communication tends to be downward. Of course, for plans to be effective and meaningful, they must not only "cascade" down the organisation from board level to every employee within the trust, but also translate into terms that can be understood by the "workers at the coal face". Much of the final service delivery is provided increasingly by external companies, so it is important that this understanding extends across both internal and external personnel. Simplicity and a common language are keys to making this work.

The likelihood of success, however, will be greater if all those who will ultimately have responsibility for delivering the end results are involved in the planning process. The best ideas are not restricted to senior managers; many of the most dramatic improvements to an organisation's processes have been suggested by operational personnel.

The power of this approach becomes apparent when the business context and strategic plans are shared with the whole organisation. This includes key external suppliers, who may deliver the majority of services. Suppliers normally focus purely on operational delivery but, when the concept of "business fundamentals" is shared, they become aware of their role in the overall planning process and are more able to contribute to tactical planning.

In the context of the internal market, external suppliers have experience which trusts do not have. They already operate in a competitive world and have developed strategies around customer-relationship management, marketing and product development. By sharing their expertise and experience, regardless of the service contracted from them, their contribution can become truly strategic for the trust.

Different skills are needed throughout a trust for working in an internal market; support and resources to make these changes have to be built into the planning process. The change itself is likely to be daunting – more so to the trust employee than to the external contractor who already lives in an uncertain world. By treating contractors and employees equally, however, it is possible to create a mutually supportive working environment.

Investment appraisal

The facilities business plan sets out objectives for performance and service over a specified period and identifies the resources and any investment required to meet those objectives. However, any organisation is likely to have more viable opportunities for investment than it has money to spend. It should therefore carry out an investment appraisal to decide where and how to invest its money to its best advantage.

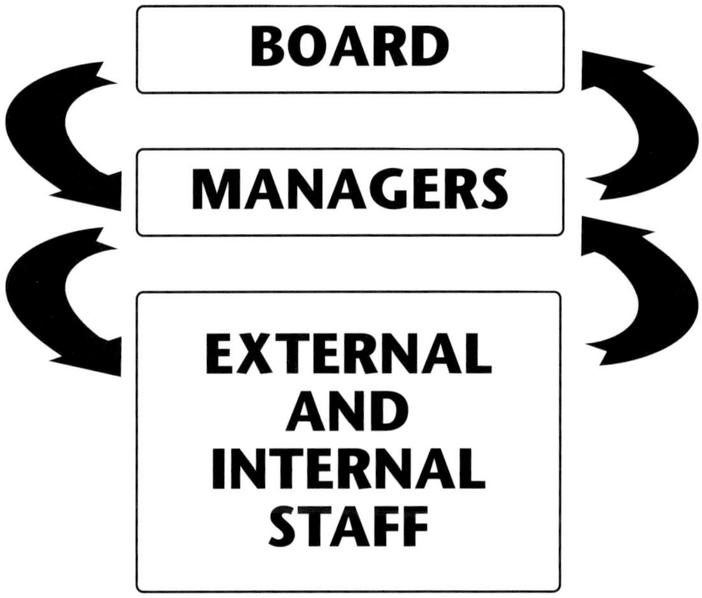

Figure 5: The two-way communication process

The objectives of investment appraisal are:

- to determine which investments make the best use of available money;
- to ensure optimum benefits from any investment made;
- to minimise the risk from making investments;
- to provide a basis for subsequent analysis of the performance of the investment.

Facilities managers should be aware of the factors which need to be taken into account in any appraisal exercise. The business case process outlined in the 'Capital Investment Manual' requires overall project investment to be assessed on a life-cycle costing basis. For example, if an organisation acquires a new building, it commits itself to a stream of costs that will be realised throughout the life of the building. These include the costs of the acquisition itself, all operation and maintenance costs, repair and replacement, alteration and improvement, ultimate replacement, recycling or disposal. These cost elements are illustrated in Figure 6. The life-cycle costing process ensures long-term value for money and guards against the danger of underfunding which may result in low health and safety standards, backlog maintenance and premature obsolescence.

The funding of life-cycle costs requires commitment of capital and revenue expenditure from different sources and under separate control in most organisations. Facilities managers should rethink the balance between capital and revenue expenditure and the traditional ways of treating buildings as fixed assets or as an overhead expense. This requires an inclusive financial package. The objectives of FM would be promoted by treating facilities as a variable rather than fixed cost of business.

The Private Finance Initiative (PFI) addresses these issues and creates new opportunities for implementation of these key concepts in the public sector. PFI promotes the application of concepts such as life-cycle costing, total cost of ownership and promises financial conditions in which FM can really develop to its full potential.

The principal objectives of PFI are to:

- transfer risk;
- promote consideration of whole life costs;
- encourage ongoing relationship between builders and maintainers;
- promote a cost-effective FM approach through centralised services.

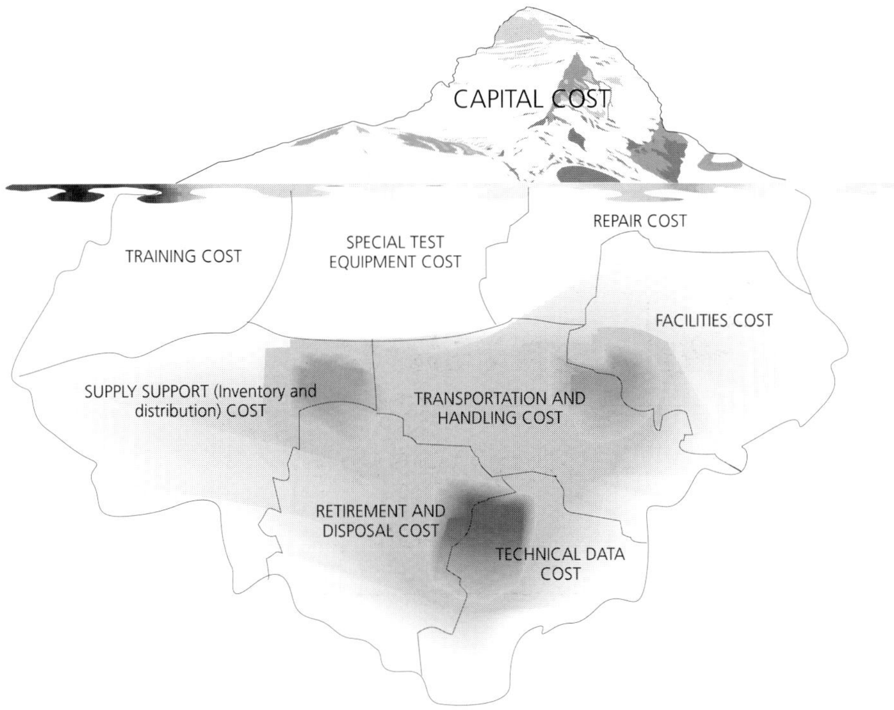

Figure 6: Life cycle costing

Assessing the financial risks associated with development, construction and maintenance, taking into account demand, performance and asset value is central to the process of developing the funding proposals. A functional risk analysis should be conducted and a weighted transfer of the risks identified should be proposed. The analysis should consider not only the risks associated with utilisation, building performance, environmental performance and operating costs but also the effects of technological change and the impact of disasters and other emergencies.

Marketing

As the focus on working for patients continues to create a service-oriented approach in the healthcare market, and further choice is introduced, internal and external marketing is becoming increasingly important. Facilities managers should market their activities to raise awareness and heighten their profile.

Marketing should be a continual process, from identifying needs through to service results and appraisal. The full range of techniques used in negotiating needs, requesting services and lodging complaints, and assessing the quality of services, creates the necessary two-way communication amongst providers and users.

Many facilities organisations in the private sector are becoming increasingly customer-oriented and are attempting to optimise the match between the demand and supply of facilities services. Marketing is essential for such a customer-oriented approach and most of these organisations have a clear "facilities marketing plan". At Schipol Airport, for example, the FM business unit provides a catalogue of products and services, so that customers can choose those which suit their operations.

This type of marketing approach requires an account manager to be appointed on behalf of the customer to act as the "informed buyer" of services and to mediate between the supplier and the customer.

Promotion and public relations are important aspects of marketing. They can help to:

- raise awareness of the importance of FM in achieving healthcare objectives;

- market facilities services within the trust;
- demonstrate value-for-money to senior management;
- publicise achievements in FM outside the organisation.

Public relations is something most of us do without thinking – that is we try to present a favourable image to the world. Internal public relations means keeping the workforce informed and involved. Focus groups and regular meetings between management and staff can help to maintain good communication. It may also be appropriate to use the media to publicise the trust's FM activities, particularly where they directly impact on public concerns for the environment and employment, and impinge on the overall reputation of the trust.

Information systems

Conventional financial accounts do not make visible the benefits of FM; most organisations are only interested in the "bottom line" or how much of a profit or loss each department is making. This is a key reason why facilities managers have had difficulty in the past in maintaining interest and commitment from senior management.

Designing a good information system involves considering the whole process of adequate data input, sensible analysis and appropriate reporting. The objective should be to reduce the amount of data that decision-makers receive whilst increasing the quality of relevant information at their disposal. Instead of producing streams of data, a system should monitor, analyse and produce output tailored for different types of decision.

The questions to ask when reviewing an existing information system are:

- who has an interest in the information it produces?
- what are they interested in knowing?
- are they getting the right information in the form that is most useful?

It is now widely accepted that information needs to be accurate, timely and relevant. But of these three requirements, the most important is relevance; information has to be appropriate to the decision to be made.

There are three levels of decision making in organisations which demand different types of information:

1. operational control;
2. managerial control;
3. strategic planning.

Information	Operational control	Managerial control	Strategic planning
Source	internal	internal	external
Precision	high	medium	low
Timing	exceptional	periodic	irregular
Notice	sudden	anticipated	none
Nature	warning	results	predictive

Table 2: Levels of decision making

Information systems should always be accurate in terms of the data gathered and information generated. The degree of precision – the variation that can be tolerated in a measurement – will vary depending on the decision to be made.

Operational decision-makers require alarms when something goes wrong, supported by precise and instant information. Managers will need periodic reports on performance. Strategic planning, however, requires two kinds of information:

- straightforward annual summary information that corresponds to a yearly review;
- information that is needed irregularly, but often urgently, to support a line of speculative enquiry.

With rare exceptions, information systems have failed to assist this kind of strategic decision-making. This failure is due to the nature of strategic decision-making which needs relatively coarse information across an unpredictably wide range of sources. Most databases do not include sufficiently wide-ranging information on all the factors that strategic decision-making might need to take into account, nor can they gather and analyse the necessary data quickly enough to be of any real use.

The NHS has well developed information systems and central returns which need to be maintained for administrative and statutory reasons. 'Estatecode', embodied in the exemplar estates strategy recommended by NHS Estates, provides such a process for property appraisal and strategic planning. The challenge is to relate facilities performance indicators to high level strategic indicators – such as occupied bed days or finished patient episodes – to provide quality business information.

C. Tactical level

Quality management

Facilities management promotes a continual improvement in the quality of the working environment and in the quality of support services at best cost. In the past, quality has been seen as an issue applicable primarily to the manufacturing sector. The service sector has been slow to recognise the advantages of introducing systems of controlling and improving quality and even today, some service providers see quality as either a low priority or even inapplicable to their business. However, attitudes to quality are now changing within many service sector organisations, particularly within the public sector. In the NHS, the Patients' Charter sets out national standards for health services. The standards are clearly defined and relatively easy to measure, leaving no ambiguity about what has to be achieved.

Total quality management

In the industrial manufacturing sector the application of Total Quality Management (TQM) has significantly improved product quality as well as reducing waste and costs to levels previously thought impossible. Such organisations have accepted the need to improve quality and, as a consequence, have improved overall market share and profit margins.

Similarly, organisations in the service sector have developed quality strategies which have assisted in the implementation of change and also empowered employees to provide a service designed to meet the needs of customers.

Many organisations have introduced regular focus groups as a way of bringing together a range of employees to discuss how quality could be improved. However, many quality initiatives fail primarily because of lack of commitment from senior management and it is estimated that 80% of organisations which commence the process of accreditation for ISO 9000 fail to reach the point at which they are sufficiently advanced to apply for registration.

Improving quality is not about increasing the number of inspections, as the inspection process simply identifies low standards of quality but does little to address the underlying cause. Improved quality is more likely to be achieved where staff are empowered to make decisions about the nature and standards of their own work.

Like many other public sector organisations, the NHS has adopted the concept of TQM although its application is variable throughout the service. The most important quality measure for customers of the NHS is the outcome of the medical treatment they receive. Whilst most users of NHS clinical services have some difficulty in determining whether the medical treatment they receive is of a high quality, they can, in most cases, make a judgment on the quality of non-clinical support services. This means users' perceptions of hospitals are often based on factors such as the quality of food, the state of decoration or the condition of the landscaping, rather than on clinical outcomes. Clearly, the areas managed within a facilities directorate have an important role to play in ensuring that a hospital offers a welcoming environment in which its activities are seen to be designed around the needs of its service users.

Introducing a TQM programme into a facilities directorate will mean:

- identifying key problem areas and applying remedial action until zero defect level is achieved;
- training employees to use new procedures;
- developing effective measures of service quality;
- creating incentives linked to quality goals;
- developing feedback mechanisms to ensure continuous improvements;
- achieving a recognised quality award, for example Charter Mark Award.

Fundamental to the success of any quality initiative is the need for good communications with both customers and staff. The starting point is accepting the need for change; for this to happen, it is essential to provide relevant information, have good operational practices and generate interest, ideas and awareness through a two-way communication process. Many organisations which introduce TQM fail to communicate effectively with their staff, as a consequence of which some promising developments fail, leading to a loss of general interest and a decline in standards of quality.

Self-assessment

Self-assessment is used by trusts to identify clearly their strengths and those areas where improvements can be made. It is also an effective means to co-ordinate quality initiatives such as ISO 9002, Investors in People, and Charter Marks.

The benefits to trusts undertaking self-assessment include:

- development of clear, concise action plans;
- clear and more focused leadership;
- better and more focused policy and strategy;
- process improvement enabling achievement of an organisation's objectives;
- improved prioritisation of resources;
- greater motivation and satisfaction of an organisation's personnel.

A self-assessment checklist is provided in Appendix I.

Team working

Fundamental to the implementation of effective quality management is the development of team working. While the strength of a team comes from the synergy it generates, it is individuals who make up the team. The first stage in introducing team working into an organisation is the development of the individual.

HFN 16 states that because facilities managers are often chosen for their skills and functional role rather than for the extent to which they complement an existing group, their team function may sometimes be overlooked. The role of the facilities manager and his/her team should be emphasised in creating the environment in which teams work. Figure 7 indicates the key roles required to make an effective team.

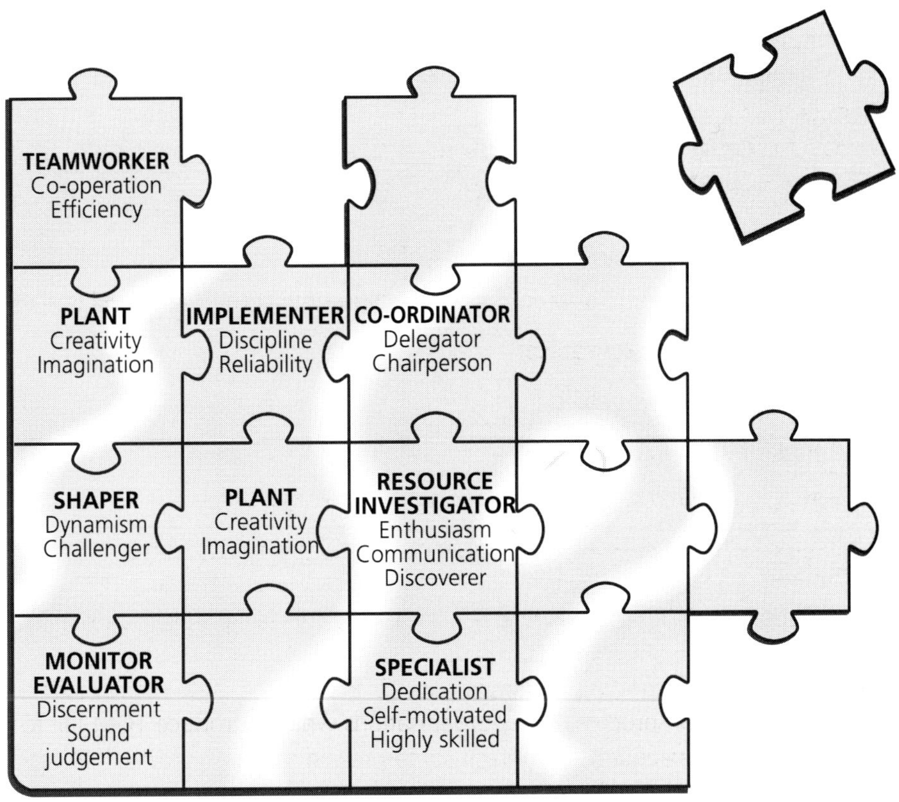

Figure 7: Key team members

In their book 'Organisational development through teambuilding', Mike Woodcock and David Francis state that an effective team will show the following characteristics:

- it will establish and work towards clear objectives;
- it will have open relationships between members;
- it will deal with different viewpoints and gain from debate;
- members will show a high level of support for each other;
- personal relationships will be based on personal knowledge and trust;
- people will want to work together and get things done;
- potentially damaging conflicts will be worked through and resolved;
- procedures and decision-making processes will be effective;
- leadership will be skillful and appropriate to the needs of the team;
- it will regularly review its operations and try to learn from experiences;

- individuals will be developed and the team will be capable of dealing with strong and weak personalities;
- relations with other groups will be co-operative and open.

However, teams may be ineffective for a variety of reasons including:

- poor selection and recruitment of team members;
- confused organisational structure;
- lack of control of the team leader;
- poor training of team members;
- low motivation;
- low creativity in team members;
- an inappropriate management philosophy;
- lack of succession planning and development;
- unclear aims;
- unfair or inappropriate rewards;
- personal stagnation in team members or leader.

Empowerment

Integral to the development of individual employees in a quality managed NHS trust is empowerment. The practice of empowerment has evolved over recent years as a means of tapping the tremendous potential that is held by an organisation's employees. The empowered workplace is characterised by:

- enhancing the content of the work;
- expanding the skills and tasks that make up the job;
- liberating creativity and innovation;
- exercising greater control over decisions about work;
- completing a whole task rather than merely portions of it;
- achieving customer satisfaction;
- developing a marketplace orientation.

Thus the empowered workplace is characterised by an environment where employer and employee are perceived as partners.

Risk will be a factor for managers deciding whether to delegate and empower. If the front line workforce is not empowered, then the emerging service-sensitive customers (internal or external) will not be satisfied. Training, qualifications and skill development must be addressed if employees are to be capable of responding to customer needs. The approach required is one of developing a learning organisation by the development of the individual as well as the organisation.

Generic working

Generic working can be defined as the provision of human resources trained to deliver a wide range of services in order to suit the needs of a particular customer group. It implies the creation of new roles which did not exist before and developing people for these roles. The principle is now well established and requires a new set of skills based on customer care and quality. The wide range of tasks requires a multi-skilled approach that cuts across several functions.

Traditionally the service sector of industry has followed a model based upon the task to be carried out. This model has created a culture organised around the needs of particular skill categories and job definitions, and has defined areas of demarcation between one discipline and another. Today that "task focused" model is obsolete as it inevitably leads to a degradation in the quality of service that can be delivered.

Trusts now need to change their approach to become customer-focused. This change in attitude must permeate all levels of the organisation from top management to front line staff. It means that staff must recognise who their particular customers are, what their needs are and must become more tuned to "on the spot" problem solving. It is necessary to recognise the diverse range of tasks required to satisfy the needs of each customer and to ensure the organisation is structured to deliver the right combination at the right time.

The design of healthcare buildings will need to reflect this new philosophy. For example, patient-focused hospital designs aim to minimise the transportation of patients between physically distant departments. The necessary facilities are provided throughout the hospital building adjacent to the patient in a unit that is staffed by multi-skilled staff trained to deliver all of the services required.

Multi-skilling

Multi-skilling may be defined as "the process of enhancing the skill repertoire of workers in such a way as to improve the ability of an employee to work in more than one narrowly defined occupational speciality" (Cordery, 1989). In other words, training people to perform two or more traditionally separate roles. Whilst this is a good general definition, to gain maximum benefit from multi-skilling it should be deep rooted rather than a skills extension programme.

Research undertaken by Akhlaghi and Mahony (1997) illustrates the benefits of multi-skilling in terms of cost and quality through studies of major schemes implemented by NHS trusts. They state: "Multi-skilling leads to increased labour flexibility and can thus reduce labour costs and increase productivity. This is because fewer spares are needed to cover absence, holiday and staff turnover. Increasing its pool of skills gives an organisation greater flexibility in its allocation of labour costs to tasks, thereby improving overall efficiency."

The organisational benefits of multi-skilling and generic working are:

- improvements in the quality of service delivered to patients;
- improvements in the continuity of service to patients;
- quicker response to meet customer need;
- reduced need to employ temporary (agency) staff;
- reduced staff absence rates.

The advantages to staff who become multi-skilled are:

- empowerment with wider responsibilities;
- greater job satisfaction;
- greater variety of work;
- opportunity to obtain qualifications (NVQs);
- opportunity for career development;
- increased pay (sometimes).

The following list is based on Akhlaghi and Mahony's (1997) list of practical steps for the implementation of a successful multi-skilling or generic working scheme:

- have a clear objective, then make this the mission for all the staff;
- network with other trusts who have implemented similar schemes;
- obtain support from the trust board;
- produce a full business plan;
- ensure that funds are identified to carry out plans;
- encourage support from staff and trade unions;
- identify training needs and ensure that these are met;
- get public relations right.

Value management

Value can be described as the achievement of the necessary function at minimum cost whilst maintaining quality, reliability and good performance. Assessing the value of a service, however, cannot be achieved without accurate methods of measuring performance. Facilities managers must have access to a range of data in order to make informed decisions about the future development of services and to react flexibly to the changing needs of the trust.

Benchmarking

Benchmarking is emerging as a powerful tool to assist facilities managers. It is used primarily for measuring costs but can also help to improve areas such as environmental practice, customer or client satisfaction, flexibility and responsiveness.

The collection of data for benchmarking can be a time consuming activity and any measurements made must therefore be relevant. The measurements employed should concentrate on areas that can add value to the business, by reducing costs or improving processes.

The individual facilities manager must decide what his/her benchmarking goals are and whether low benchmark costs are of value or not. There is an inevitable cycle to "cost only benchmarking": as costs are driven down, initially from improved processes and practices, the scope for improvement will decrease and reduced quality may be the result.

When using benchmarking as a tool, whether for cost or process improvements, it is important that "like for like" comparisons are made. Comparing the security system in an inner city hospital with security in a rural community hospital, for example, will be of little use unless the differences are recognised and appropriate adjustments made. The data on which the benchmarking system is based (accurate drawings and calculations of space) are established and agreed with all stakeholders. Although a number of benchmarking "clubs" or databases are emerging, the way in which the information is used or analysed differs from one healthcare organisation to another. There would, therefore, appear to be scope for the development of a standardised approach.

Example

An acute trust adopted regression analysis as the basis for examining the data supplied by a benchmarking club. Key performance indicators were selected and the data relating to other similar trusts was expressed graphically as a "line of best fit" between cost/m^2 and size in m^2. The trust's own values were plotted to indicate variance from the norm value. Those indicators with wide variance were then investigated to identify reasons for the differences, identify targets for improvement and set action plans.

In its document 'Costing models for FM performance' the Health Estates Facilities Management Association (HEFMA) concludes that the purpose of measuring costs is to:

- provide data for planning purposes;
- track existing service delivery costs.

Performance benchmarking is considered to be the most useful "tool" available to the facilities manager. HEFMA suggests that if analysis is based on the cost of occupancy, using fixed and variable components, this will align FM with business planning. It also believes that the ability to break down costs to centres within the trust extends the benefits that can be gained from benchmarking.

Performance measurement

The British Institute of Facilities Management (BIFM, 1995) recommends the following key FM business ratios and measures.

Facilities/turnover ratio	Total annual cost of facilities as a proportion of total annual turnover.
Facilities/profit ratio	Total annual cost of facilities as a proportion of gross annual profit.
Facilities/sales ratio	Total annual cost of facilities as a proportion of total annual sales revenues.
Facilities/asset ratio	Total annual cost of facilities as a proportion of total fixed asset value.
Facilities utilisation	Number of hours per week facilities in actual use as a proportion of total number of hours in a week.
Facilities/staff ratio	Total annual cost of facilities as a proportion of total annual staff costs.

Other indicators may include:

Facilities/operating costs ratio	Total annual cost of facilities as a proportion of total operating costs of the organisation.
	This ratio indicates the significance of facilities costs. In commercial office settings this may be 13% of the organisation's operating costs, while in healthcare settings it can be more than 35% (or more if capital charges are included).
Facilities/revenue ratio	Total annual cost of facilities as a proportion of the revenue associated with the use of particular facilities.

This will enable exploration of opportunity costs.

Risk management

The NHS Management Executive has confirmed that the management of risk must be accepted by all NHS managers as one of their key responsibilities. Risk management can be defined as the identification, analysis and economic control of those risks which can threaten the assets or earning capacity of an enterprise.

Corporate risk management is concerned with the approach an organisation adopts to minimise risk exposure. Developing a corporate risk management policy entails:

- considering the impact of all risks that could affect the trust's business;
- developing strategies that control these risks within the framework of the trust's mission and risk management philosophy;
- monitoring, reviewing and revising strategies to ensure the trust maintains competitive advantage.

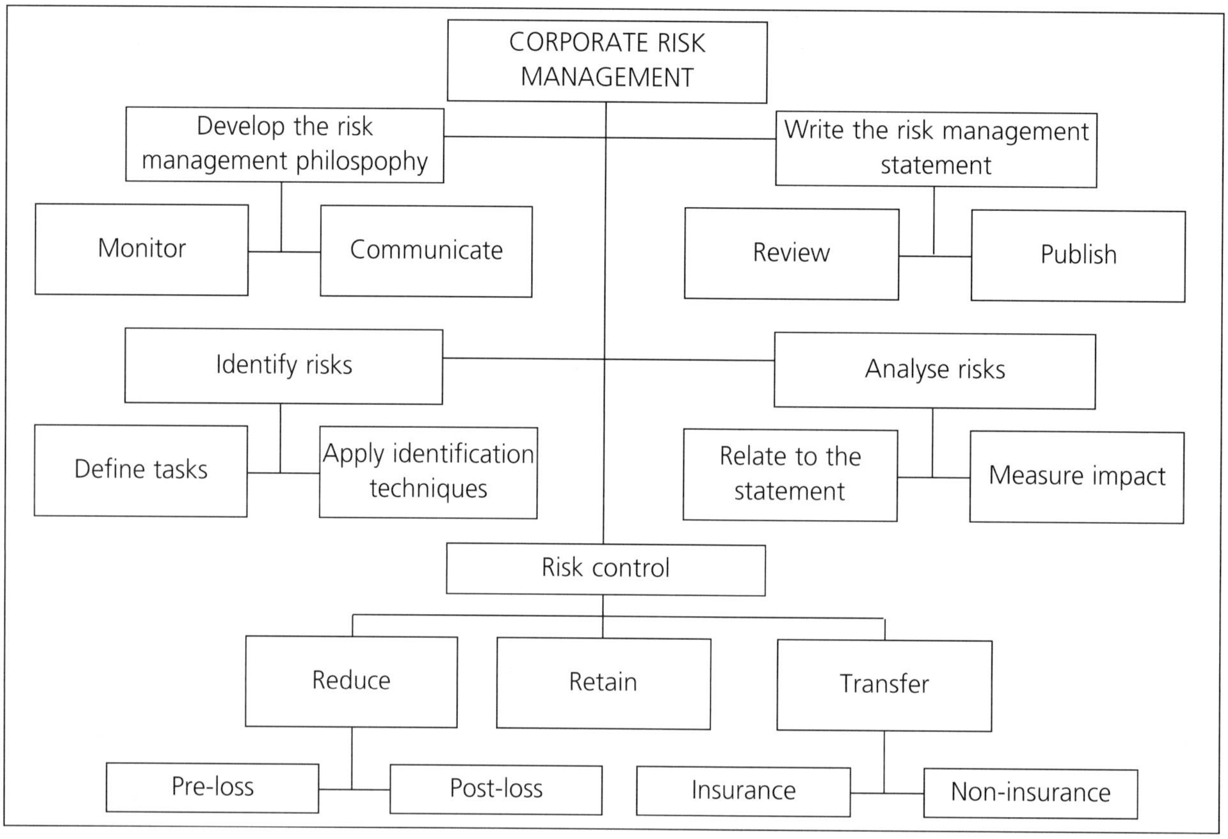

Figure 8: The risk management process

Acting as the interface between staff and the workplace, facilities managers are arguably best positioned to take the lead in developing a corporate risk management strategy. Although the risk management policy should ultimately be set by the trust board, all disciplines at strategic, tactical and operational levels should be involved in formulating the strategy. This will ensure a holistic approach. It is recommended that a risk management committee is formed where the various disciplines, including facilities management, can be represented. Communication is a key factor in developing a risk management culture.

As well as contributing to the corporate risk management process, facilities managers will need to focus on the risk management of individual FM services.

Security

Security measures to reduce the risks of vandalism, theft, attacks on staff and patients, the abduction of babies from maternity units and a range of other problems may be operational or physical. Operational measures include requiring staff to conform to security procedures, training them in crime prevention techniques, and contracting a professional security firm to provide surveillance. Physical controls include staff identification systems, the installation of closed circuit television, intruder alarms, electronic tagging of infants, digital locks and key control systems. Risk assessment can help to identify the most cost-effective solutions to security problems.

Fire safety

One of the major problems in the NHS is the backlog of work that needs to be undertaken to ensure that the estate meets the required fire safety standards. Trusts will need to carry out risk assessments to identify the hazards and calculate risk exposures. This will enable them to establish priorities so that improvement programmes can be agreed and accounted for in business plans.

The private finance initiative (PFI) has implications for fire safety in hospitals. Novel design solutions appearing as a result of PFI are not necessarily required to comply with 'Firecode' but should demonstrate an equal level of fire safety. In addition, the contracting-out of facilities management services can result in ill-defined fire evacuation responsibilities of trust and contracted-out staff. All PFI proposals and service contracts should adequately address the issue of fire safety.

Buildings, equipment and plant

As for fire safety, one of the major problems for existing premises is the backlog of building maintenance work. If repairs are extensive, budgets may not be large enough to fund all the necessary work. In such cases, a list of priorities must be established through risk assessment. In new buildings, a planned preventive maintenance programme can be more cost-effective than carrying out repairs at a later date. If asbestos is present in the building, its type, condition and extent should be recorded so that risks to people working in the area can be minimised. Water supplies also present particular hazards: a named individual should be responsible for precautions against legionella.

Waste disposal

All trusts are responsible for ensuring that waste materials are correctly disposed of. Unsafe practices may result in high risk to patients, staff, the public in general and the environment, and can lead to heavy fines.

Section 34 of The Environmental Protection Act 1990 'Waste management – the duty of care, a code of practice' should be used as a benchmark of good practice. It requires waste to be properly segregated and labelled, securely stored and transferred, and places the responsibility for ensuring safe disposal at a licensed site firmly with the producer of the waste.

The costs of waste removal are rising, as the incineration of clinical waste is strictly licensed, and bulk non-clinical waste going to landfill is subject to taxation. Advice on clinical waste management is contained in HTM 2065 – 'Healthcare waste management', 'A strategic guide to clinical waste management' (NHS Estates), HGN – 'Clinical waste incineration: Joint venture arrangements', and HGN – 'Safe disposal of clinical waste: Whole hospital guidance'.

Health and safety

Health and safety management will be an important aspect of a facilities manager's role. 'The Management of the Health and Safety at Work Regulations' requires employers to carry out a systematic assessment of workplace risks and, as a consequence, to put into place preventive and protective measures, in the form of a health and safety strategy.

A successful strategy depends on accurate reporting systems, effective communication and appropriate training for staff. The Health and Safety Executive's booklet 'Successful health and safety management' sets out a framework for developing a pro-active management system, including setting clear objectives and auditing performance.

Reputation risk management

Facilities managers are increasingly having to consider the management of reputation risk. This is a difficult task as reputation is based on people's perceptions, which will vary widely. For reputation risk management to be implemented effectively, managers need to understand the organisational culture and how individual's perceptions are shaped. The general risk management principles of identification, analysis and control should be applied to reputation risk.

D. Operational level

Operational planning

Having defined the strategic breakthrough plan for the year, and the infrastructure needed to support it, there is also a need to ensure that the day-to-day business is kept on track. This is done by setting a small number of key measurement indicators, known as the "business fundamentals", that indicate if something is going wrong. A range of typical indicators is listed in Table 3.

Estate costs:
Facilities costs as a percentage of revenue
Maintenance costs per square metre
Non-attendance days per employee
Planned preventive maintenance hours per square metre
Mean time between plant failures

Catering:
Average cost per patient day
Main meal equivalent production per operative
Level of wastage as a percentage of total (raw material value)

Transport:
Maintenance cost per mile
Cost of ownership per mile

Linen:
Cleaning cost per garment
Repairs as a percentage of total throughput

Miscellaneous:
Level of complaints against activity level
Response time to requests/complaints
Customer satisfaction

Table 3: Typical performance indicators

For each fundamental, targets and measures are set. Performance against business fundamentals takes the form of a traffic light system – red for off-track, amber for not-on-target but within acceptable parameters, and green for on-track. This allows a manager to see at a glance how things are going on a day-to-day basis. These are then reviewed on a monthly basis and the results rolled-up to the next management level for broader departmental or company review.

The same review format is applied to the implementation plans supporting the key strategies. These are reviewed quarterly and prompt the documentation of corrective action should a strategy start going off-track. All too often, sound planning is done and then ignored until the next planning period. Business changes in the meantime may well have negated aspects of the plan, so a constant review is essential, and flexibility needs to be built into the facilities plans. Scenario planning, another recognised business tool, can help to predict the "unexpected".

3.0 The case studies

Introduction

The five trusts studied in this chapter illustrate FM practice in a range of acute, community and mental health trusts. They have been selected to represent different aspects of and stages in the development of FM, and are not intended to be exemplars of best practice.

Blackpool Victoria Hospital NHS Trust

The following case study identifies some of the challenges of introducing FM at Blackpool Victoria Hospital and demonstrates what has been achieved since the directorate was formed. These benefits include an improvement in the quality of services delivered whilst achieving annual savings in excess of £500,000.

Trust mission statement

Victoria Hospital has developed a reputation as a customer focused organisation and the additional independence since the assumption of trust status has provided the opportunity to further improve the quality of the services provided. The philosophy of the trust is summed up in its mission statement:

'To provide the highest quality of care to our patients in the most cost effective way.'

Trust profile

Number of beds	764 on main site 92 contracted from adjoining community trust
Number of patients	45,000 in-patients 18,000 day cases 54,800 out patients 81,000 A&E patients each year
Number of staff	2,386 whole time equivalents
Size of site	14.2 hectares
Total floor area	81,000 m^2
Current value of the estate	£56 million
Annual income	£75.8 million
FM budget	£9.3 million

Background

The Blackpool Victoria Hospital NHS Trust was formed in April 1994. It is a busy acute unit which is one of four regional cardiology and cardiothoracic centres in the North West.

In addition to providing healthcare for a resident population of 320,000 people (many of whom are retired) the trust also provides a service to 18 million tourists who visit the resort each year.

Situated approximately 1½ miles from Blackpool town centre the buildings on site are an assortment of varying ages and architectural styles, which range from the original buildings of the 1930s to present day modern developments.

Nine of the wards currently operational were built to accommodate emergency medical services during the second world war, and were expected to have a maximum life of five to 10 years. Approval has now been given to replace these buildings through a major capital redevelopment of the site, completion of which is programmed for the end of the century.

Corporate level

Development of facilities management services

Prior to the assumption of trust status, the responsibility for non-clinical support services at Victoria Hospital was shared amongst seven senior managers. Such fragmentation of management arrangements made it difficult to achieve a customer focused approach to some services.

At the inception of the trust, it was decided that all non-clinical support services would be provided by a single directorate, the anticipated benefits of which were:

- single point of contact for service users;
- increased flexibility of resources;
- development of a team approach amongst staff;
- elimination of duplication of effort;
- improved customer care;
- improved development opportunities for staff;
- delivery of more cost-effective services.

An integrated FM directorate was created comprising all non-clinical support services.

The directorate's revenue budget for 1996-97 was £9.3 million. It is also responsible for managing an annual capital programme in excess of £7 million.

The majority of non-clinical support services are delivered by in-house staff although cleaning services (with an annual value of £1.2 million) are outsourced. Similarly, all capital developments and the majority of major maintenance work is competitively tendered and provided by the private sector.

Facilities management organisational structure

The directorate currently employs 323 whole time equivalent staff (which equates to 13.5% of the total employed by the trust). The management structure is shown in Figure 9.

Facilities management mission statement

The trust recognises that in the delivery of high quality healthcare the quality of its non-clinical support services is an important factor in the general public's perceptions of the total organisation. As most customers form an opinion of an organisation within a few minutes of arriving on site, to create the most favourable impression of Blackpool Victoria Hospital the following factors were considered important:

- ease of access to the site;
- ease of parking on the site;
- quality of signposting;
- ease of access to buildings;
- provision of appropriate facilities for disabled people;
- layout and maintenance of grounds and gardens.

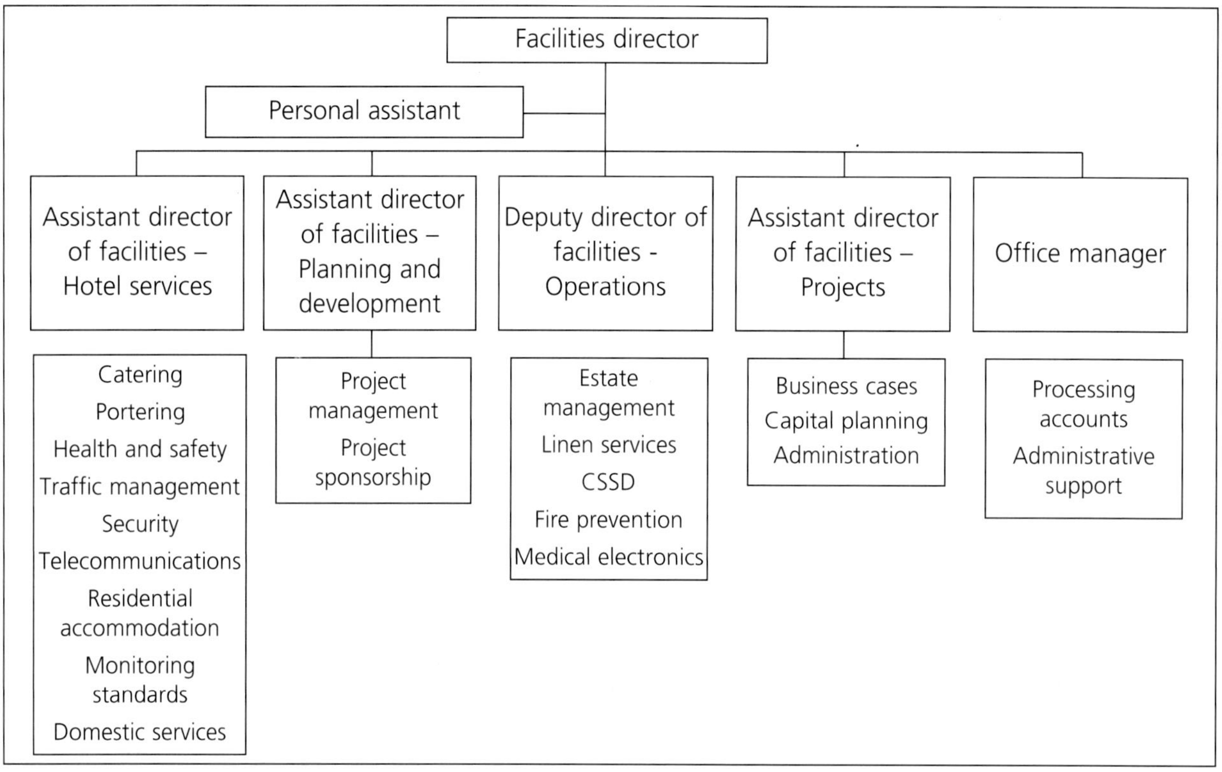

Figure 9: Facilities directorate structure

The FM directorate was charged with ensuring that the above issues were properly addressed and in order to do so it was considered necessary to develop a directorate mission statement to complement the trust's philosophy.

FM mission statement

The vision
To be the best and most successful FM directorate in the healthcare sector.

The strategy
Our strategy to achieve the vision is:

- To exceed our customers' expectations by delivering support services of a high quality in a professional manner, on time and within agreed costs.
- To constantly seek to improve quality standards and efficiency in all areas of our activities.
- To recognise and respect individual contribution whilst providing and promoting opportunities for personal growth and development.

The values
To deliver our strategy:

- We will use the vitality, commitment and skill of our staff to provide a foundation for our continual success.
- We will build on this strength by encouraging teamworking and employee involvement in all aspects of our activities.
- We will provide effective leadership and behave with clarity, trust and openness at all times.

Through training, informal discussions, roadshows and team briefings, staff are continually reminded of the directorate's mission statement and are encouraged to challenge the current methods of delivering non-clinical support services. This approach reflects the philosophy of the trust which has developed a culture where staff are encouraged to maximise their full potential, organisational barriers are removed, and team working is promoted at all levels.

Strategic level

Strategic direction

In a climate of change for the delivery of healthcare the following factors have to be taken into account when developing a strategy for the future:

- the shift from secondary to primary care;
- the total allocation (and distribution) of funding for the provision of healthcare services;
- the concept and development of GP fundholding;
- the impact of private finance initiatives;
- the non-availability of NHS capital funding;
- the requirement to market test services.

Following extensive consultations with purchasers, other providers and a range of interest groups, the trust's strategic direction document was developed to reflect these factors. It establishes a framework for the delivery of support services which includes a commitment to continually and radically review the delivery of services to ensure that they complement the trust's business objectives at all times.

The strategy identifies short, medium and long-term objectives for each department together with the capital investment necessary to achieve those objectives.

Business plan and marketing strategy

The facilities strategy is supported by an annual business plan which follows a similar format to the strategic direction document and identifies the objective for each department for the planning period. The document incorporates action plans and is subject to quarterly reviews by senior managers within the directorate.

The directorate recently compiled a marketing strategy for its key departments. The strategy establishes a framework for marketing its services and identifies the individual approach that will be pursued by each department. It also identifies key tasks and performance targets which are subject to regular monitoring by senior facilities managers.

As competition for the delivery of healthcare services increases, the pressure to reduce costs to a minimum will inevitably grow. In this environment, the delivery of support services must remain flexible and complement the trust's business objectives. Support service providers have access to a range of complementary documents similar to those identified above so they are familiar with the trust's strategic direction.

Provision of services to other trusts and the private sector

The majority of services provided by the directorate are supplied exclusively to the trust although, increasingly, the directorate is selling its surplus capacity to other trusts, through service level agreements, and the private sector through normal commercial practices. The linen services department has been particularly successful in selling its services to the private sector, and in the last three years has increased its annual turnover to private customers from £15,000 to over £200,000. The recent achievement of ISO 9002 provides an opportunity for a further expansion of the service into the private sector which is planned to increase by £50,000 a year.

Tactical level

Customer care

The directorate recognises that to retain customers it is essential to provide good quality services and it was necessary to gain the commitment of all staff to promote a friendly, helpful image. The starting point was the development of a customer care charter:

Customer care charter

Our vision is to be the best and most successful FM directorate in the healthcare sector.

We promise to provide the most efficient and cost effective service to our customers by adopting the following principles:

- Putting the customer first at all times.
- Providing a friendly, helpful service delivered by well trained staff.
- Listening to our customers and dealing swiftly with complaints.
- Delivering competitive, high quality, innovative services.
- Being sensitive to the needs of our customers.
- Creating a culture that recognises achievement and encourages ownership.
- Seeking continuous improvements in all our activities.
- Providing our employees with job satisfaction and the opportunity for personal development.

An intensive interactive training programme was developed for all staff. Customer care surveys were introduced to determine customer requirements and to identify better ways to anticipate and fulfil them.

Customers were asked to rate the service as excellent, very good, adequate or poor. Where ratings are poor or adequate the departmental manager investigates with the customer, takes the appropriate action and reports back to the FM director. The results of the customer care surveys are made available to all customers and regular reports are presented to the trust board identifying the outcome. Managers are encouraged to deal with complaints swiftly and efficiently. However, if a customer remains dissatisfied with a particular service, they have direct access to the FM director.

Customer surveys have an important role to play in determining views on the quality of services delivery. However, it would be naive to believe that they are a completely accurate reflection of customers' views. To complement the results of customer surveys, the FM director has regular informal meetings with all business and nurse managers. These meetings are used as a means of validating the result of the surveys and also provide an opportunity to make the customer feel valued.

Benchmarking

External benchmarking provides an opportunity for the trust to compare its support services with those of similar organisations. Having analysed the information provided by a number of benchmarking organisations, the directorate joined the Healthcare Facilities Consortium benchmarking arrangement. Information from the consortium is examined on a regular basis to determine if the services provided by the directorate can be improved.

Table 4 reveals that, in financial terms, the directorate's performance compares favourably with that of other organisations.

	Trust £ per m^2	Average costs for similar hospital £ per m^2
Total utility costs	13.58	14.26
Estate maintenance costs	12.76	13.33
Grounds and garden maintenance costs	0.37	0.48
Security costs	0.33	0.86
Insurance costs	1.03	1.83

Table 4: Benchmarking performance data

In addition to participating in the national benchmarking arrangements, the directorate is a member of a benchmarking club comprising six similar organisations. Regular meetings of the club are held and the data provided by each organisation is examined in detail to determine the reason for any variation in the cost of services. Cost is clearly important, but not the only factor in comparing services. An allowance must also be made to reflect the quality of the services delivered.

Internal benchmarking which compares current costs to those incurred during a similar period in previous years is also a useful measure of performance. The directorate has developed a number of internal benchmarks, including:

- estates maintenance cost/m^2;
- energy used GJ/m^3;
- number of meals served;
- income generated in the staff dining room;
- number of incoming telephone calls received;
- cost of processing linen per item.

To ensure that the information provided is meaningful, an adjustment is made to reflect changes in activity and other factors that might effect the validity of the data.

Environmental management

During the last few years there has been increased public and political interest in environmental issues with an increase in environmental legislation in both the UK and Europe. The trust has recognised that staff commitment to pro-environmental policies is fundamental to its success and, consequently, significant efforts are made to keeping staff informed and involved in all aspects of protecting the environment. A key environmental objective was to reduce waste by adopting the 3Rs principle:

- reduce waste;
- re-use;
- re-cycle re-usable resources.

The trust's ongoing commitment to protect the environment is detailed in its strategic direction document. Initiatives planned for the future include:

a. Meeting and exceeding all relevant national and European regulations and assisting in developing solutions to environmental problems.

b. Establishing standards where national and/or European regulations do not exist.

c. Helping to preserve natural resources by developing and implementing immediate strategies to:

- further reduce the use of water and energy;
- reduce the use of materials which originate from non-renewable sources;
- make more economical and effective use of products such as paper, glass and plastic, cans, batteries and other similar products;
- ensure the products used by the trust's staff (or its contractors) contain minimal ozone depleting substances;
- develop further strategies in relation to vehicle emissions, horticultural products, asbestos, toxic solvents, biodegradable substances, litter and many others;
- achieve BS 7750 'Specification for Environmental Management Systems'.

The trust's environmental initiatives are determined and monitored by a multi-disciplinary committee chaired by the facilities director. Initiatives already implemented include:

- creation of a wildflower meadow which attracts 11 species of butterfly;
- provision of bird nesting boxes;
- introduction of an initiative to re-cycle paper;
- issue of bicycle purchase grants in exchange for car parking permits;
- improvements to the external landscaping;
- reduction in the unnecessary use of energy and water;
- reduction in the use of unsustainable tropical hard woods;
- reduction in the use of synthetic pesticides and artificial fertilisers;
- arranging an environmental open day to encourage staff participation and awareness.

Operational level

Training and staff development

The chairman and non-executive directors are encouraged to visit support service departments to meet the operational staff and gain a greater understanding of the challenges of delivering support services in a hospital environment. This is critical to the success of the FM directorate but equally important is the need to keep staff fully informed of the achievements and challenges of the directorate. A number of projects have been organised to encourage and motivate staff:

- production of a directorate annual report;
- delivery of an annual road show;
- regular team briefings;
- staff appraisals;
- recognition of achievements;
- informal discussions;
- directorate newsletter;
- staff attitude survey.

Training and development within the directorate is delivered in a number of different ways depending on the needs of the organisation and the individuals concerned. Shadowing, mentoring and coaching are particularly encouraged. The achievement of NVQ awards for key support services staff is considered fundamental to the delivery of high quality services. A number of staff have already qualified to the appropriate standards and some have trained as appraisers for other staff.

Future developments

The challenge for the trust's FM directorate is to undertake a radical review of all aspects of the services under its control and to initiate whatever changes and improvements are necessary.

The directorate's strategy establishes a framework for the delivery of support services in the future. In the medium to long term (that is, three to five years) the FM directorate will:

- ensure that 50% of its staff are qualified to the appropriate NVQ level;
- continue to market test appropriate support services;
- radically review the delivery of support services;
- examine alternative means by which people may travel to and from hospital;
- consider the feasibility of providing hotel style services to patients;
- examine the feasibility of home working, desk sharing and neighbourhood offices.

The strategy sets out a challenging agenda for the directorate which, if achieved, will ensure the provision of high quality, cost-effective non-clinical support services which complement the healthcare activities provided by the trust.

Analysis

The trust's aims are presented as a facilities challenge. The objectives are documented and communicated in the business plan, and are supported by action plans and a marketing strategy. From this secure base, the facilities organisation can then seek opportunities to market services externally, to minimise the overhead by working to full capacity.

The trust has a strong environmental policy with initiatives determined and monitored by a multi-disciplinary committee chaired by the director of facilities. The trust recognises its responsibility to comply with environmental legislation and the need for environmental management systems designed to minimise any adverse impact on the environment which may arise from its activities.

Environment, services and "front-of-house" provision are the responsibility of the facilities management department. The Trust has a strong customer orientation and recognises the need for culture change and illustrates its commitment to this through the customer care charter, customer satisfaction surveys, quality audits and action groups.

The Hairmyres and Stonehouse Hospitals NHS Trust

This case study explores the development of facilities management (FM) at the Hairmyres and Stonehouse hospitals since becoming an NHS trust. It examines the framework that has been adopted by the new FM directorate to enable them to assess, evaluate and develop good practice and innovation in all aspects of service provision and management in a healthcare environment. Finally, it looks at future plans for a new hospital under the private finance initiative (PFI).

Trust mission statement

'To deliver high quality, efficient patient care in collaboration with the trust's purchasers and, through leadership and support, create an environment in which the trust's staff are committed to, and contribute to the trust's aims and objectives.'

The Trust aims to provide:

- more locally focused management to facilitate speedier decision making;
- increased patient choice and involvement in decision making in respect of individual care;
- better information systems and practices;
- closer liaison with GPs and local authorities;
- a more valued and motivated workforce.

Trust profile

Number of beds	(Hairmyres)	532
	(Stonehouse)	235
Number of patients 1995-96		24,401 in-patients 11,685 day cases, 29,176 new out-patients 41,836 A&E cases
Number of staff		1,460 whole time equivalents
Size of site	(Hairmyres)	32.8 hectares
	(Stonehouse)	14 hectares
Total floor area		66,534 m^2
Current value of estate	(Hairmyres)	£34.9 million
	(Stonehouse)	£7.8 million
Annual income		£49 million per annum
Capital charges		£4.6 million (£18.92/m^2)
FM budget		£13 million (including utility and supplies costs)

Background

The Hairmyres and Stonehouse Hospitals NHS Trust was formed in April 1994. Previously, Hairmyres Hospital and Stonehouse Hospital formed part of the Hamilton and East Kilbride Directly Managed Unit (DMU), one of four within Lanarkshire Health Board. The DMU comprised the following psychiatric, community and acute hospitals:

- Hairmyres Hospital;
- Stonehouse Hospital;
- Kirklands Hospital;
- Birkwood Hospital;
- Bellfield Hospital;
- Udston Hospital.
- a number of primary healthcare centres in East Kilbride and surrounding area.

It is now one of Scotland's 34 acute trusts. The remaining hospitals and health centres were transferred to the Community and Priority Services Unit of Lanarkshire Health Board, which is now the Lanarkshire Healthcare NHS Trust.

Hairmyres Hospital is located on the south west boundary of East Kilbride, some 14 miles from Stonehouse Hospital which is located in the village of Stonehouse. All of the buildings are owned by the trust. The trust has contractual leases with the Scottish Ambulance Service for the ambulance station and with Lanarkshire Healthcare trust for two psychiatric wards and the psychiatric day hospital. Hairmyres Hospital has 750 car spaces and Stonehouse has 190 car spaces.

The sites of both hospitals are fragmented in nature and were last extended during the war years when emergency medical service huts were erected. Although some extension and upgrading has taken place since then, most in-patient services are still provided within the original facilities. Because of the physical characteristics of the estate, only limited opportunities are provided for upgrading with no feasible, comprehensive solution to accommodation problems. The widely distributed layout of buildings, as well as the two site operation, present significant constraints on the cost, efficiency and quality of services. As a result of the poor physical layout of the estates, the DMU was authorised by the Management Executive in Scotland to pursue PFI funding for a new hospital at Hairmyres (see Future developments on page 42).

Corporate level

Organisational structure

The trust board comprises:

- chairman;
- 5 executive directors (including the chief executive and the FM director);
- 5 Non-Executive directors.

The trust board is responsible for determining the trust's strategic direction and monitoring operational plans and performance. The management team includes corporate and clinical directors who support the trust board and act as the link between the strategic level (corporate policy) and the operational level (service level) of the trust's structure.

Development of facilities management services

Hairmyres Hospital has a long history in the field of estate evaluation, dating from the late 1980s when it was involved in a pilot study to investigate ways of improving the efficiency and economy of estate management. The hospital's involvement in this exercise contributed to the development of effective FM tools, which were used to achieve and maintain adequate and economic standards in the condition, safety and efficiency of its physical resources. The whole process enabled the organisation to raise fundamental questions about the way in which the estate could be managed to ensure that:

- the estates department made the most of the physical resources;
- building performance data was related to investment, costs and expectancy;
- the estate was seen as an asset not a liability;
- property data was appropriately structured for effective estate management.

This introduction to FM enabled the estates department to gain valuable information and experience, which it has now been able to apply in the long term through the FM directorate of the new trust.

Facilities management organisational structure

The new organisational structure required one or two changes to be made:

- the original estates manager became the new FM director, responsible for all non-clinical support services under a unified FM structure;
- the original director of administration and support services became board secretary, responsible for the trust's corporate affairs.

The current management structure of the trust has been in place since its inception and was designed to facilitate the strategic, management and clinical service delivery functions.

Figure 10 illustrates the organisational structure of the FM directorate.

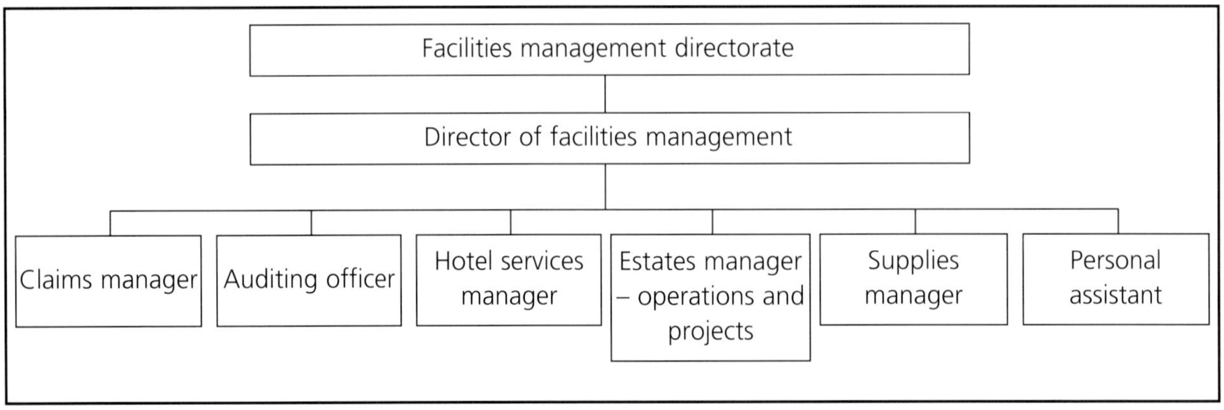

Figure 10: Facilities directorate structure

In the transition to trust status, the management and staff were faced with the challenge of adapting to the new organisational structure, culture and working practices. This is an ongoing process which has proved to be more difficult than initially anticipated. Although there is no formal strategy for FM education and training at present, the trust recognises that a staff development programme will be necessary.

Strategic level

Strategic direction

With all FM support services managed and co-ordinated by one individual accountable to the chief executive, many of the historical boundaries along with accompanying inefficiencies could be tackled. A support services auditing department was established to monitor both quality and financial performance of all FM contracts. It was also decided that health and safety management could best be undertaken by the FM director, thereby bringing together the statutory regulations and codes of practice relating to the estate and FM services with the statutory duties to employees and the public. Under this arrangement, claims management would also transfer to the FM director.

The trust sees this strategy as essential preparation for the possible move to a new hospital in the future. It recognises that the provision of healthcare within a privately owned, fully serviced building, will require specific skills and expertise which are not compatible with the traditional NHS administration and management structure.

This strategic and operational development is driven by a number of factors including:

- national priorities as defined in national guidelines;
- the need to provide quality healthcare in an efficient an effective manner;
- the requirement to operate in a competitive environment;
- the empowerment of NHS consumers;
- the relationship between the trust and the special purpose company providing healthcare in a privately owned fully serviced building.

Information management

In 1993 the DMU undertook a three-year resource management project designed to introduce new information systems to support clinicians and managers. This new approach aims to ensure that good quality information is available to support clinical and managerial staff to improve overall planning, management and delivery of services to patients.

This project enabled the trust to:

- secure new systems;
- improve current systems as necessary;
- create an integrated clinical and resource information system;
- have the IT strategy approved by the trust board.

Tactical level

Quality management

The trust is committed to providing high quality services for patients. Through investment in training initiatives, for example NVQs, the staff have become more focused on developing organisational standards. Patients' satisfaction with service delivery is monitored through a number of feedback mechanisms such as the patients' meal questionnaire which is carried out on a monthly basis. These responses are then evaluated and action taken where necessary.

The staff and management also have an opportunity to voice their opinion on the quality of services through the customer feedback form, introduced to service users in June 1996. This allows the directorate to monitor the quality of all FM services.

Other initiatives include the introduction of a call logger system to monitor the performance of the switchboard service and a telephone help desk system for FM services. The strategic management of all medical and non-electronic equipment has been established with respect to a replacement programme, the management of service contracts and their routine maintenance and repairs.

In 1995 the trust undertook its first King's Fund organisational audit (quality systems/FM systems audit; for example, patient care profiles, staff training, fire safety), enabling standards to be set for the entire range of trust activities. The audit process validated good practice and identified areas where improvements could be made, including:

- Communication: Information booklets for in-patients and out-patients have been produced and have been awarded Crystal Marks by the Plain English Campaign.
- Customer satisfaction: A marked reduction in the number of complaints received by the trust, from 198 in 1994-95 to 106 in 1995-96.

The trust received the award of accreditation during 1996, and the hospital accreditation programme's software system is now being piloted at the trust.

Value management

The practice of value management is incorporated into the organisation through the use of standardised performance indicators such as:

- Scottish Office Annual Energy Report for the Energy Performance.
- Hotel services catering costs with catering value performance indicators (weekly food costs per patient).

All budgets are carefully scrutinised, with the emphasis on achieving "value for money". Regular reviews of FM service requirements and the costs of achieving them are carried out by the Auditing Officer using the above performance indicators plus other tools including market testing, customer satisfaction surveys and past experience of the healthcare industry.

Risk management

In September 1995, as part of the King's Fund audit, the trust produced its first risk management strategy to address non-clinical risks. This was revised in March 1996 to form the corporate risk management strategy document.

A risk management committee, chaired by the FM director, is to be established to devise a practical and systematic framework for focusing the trust's approach to risk management.

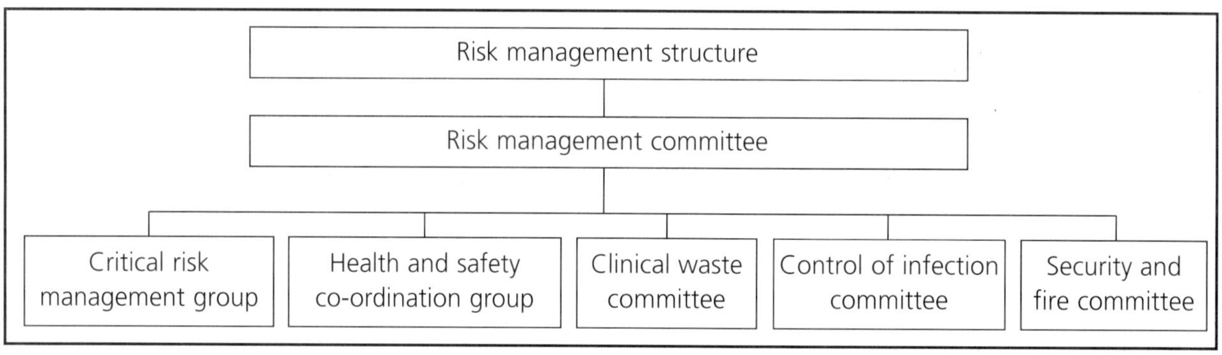

Figure 11: Risk management structure

The main aims of the new risk management strategy are:

- to improve the safety of patients, visitors, staff and others affected by the work of the trust;

- to enhance the quality of patient care;
- to minimise the trust's financial liability due to substandard patient care or unsafe conditions.

Environmental management

The trust promotes a pro-environmental regime through the use of 'Greencode', issued by the NHS in Scotland Healthcare Engineering and Environment Unit. Phase one of Greencode is currently being pilot tested at eight sites in Scotland, including Hairmyres and Stonehouse trust, and will be formally launched in 1997.

It is the trust's intention to remain committed to the use of energy efficiency measures and encourage good practice in relation to housekeeping through a programme of staff education and training. Through its links with the Healthcare Engineering and Environment Unit, the FM directorate is able to share information and experiences with others in the healthcare industry.

The Healthcare Engineering and Environment Unit and the King's Fund are looking at the possibility of using Greencode as a criteria for accreditation purposes.

Operational level

Overview of non-clinical support services

Over the last two years responsibility for the management of all non-clinical support services has been transferred to the FM director. The services include hotel, administrative and supply functions. A mixture of in-house and outsourced service contracts are provided, which are market tested with the aim of ensuring the best possible service at the lowest cost.

The trust purchases a range of services from other NHS trusts via Service Level Agreements (SLAs). It also sells a small number of services to other trusts. Over the past few years the trust has invested heavily in developing its catering and housekeeping functions, as well as the physical environment, to ensure that the patient's visit or stay is made as comfortable as possible. Table 5 lists the full range of services along with the type of contract for each service.

Non-clinical services	Hairmyres	Stonehouse
Communications	In-house	In-house
Estates management	In-house	In-house
Reception	In-house	In-house
Supplies	In-house	In-house
Catering	In-house	Outsourced
Domestic services	In-house	Outsourced
Residences	In-house	Outsourced
Estate maintenance	Outsourced	Outsourced
Painting	Outsourced	Outsourced
Parking management	Outsourced	Outsourced
Portering	Outsourced	Outsourced
Security	Outsourced	Outsourced
Transport	Outsourced	Outsourced
Clinical waste	*SLA	*SLA
CSSD/TSSU	*SLA	*SLA
IT/Computer services	*SLA	*SLA
Laundry and linen	*SLA	*SLA
Medical physics	*SLA	*SLA

* Service Level Agreements

Table 5: Contracts for non-clinical services

Service contracts can be broken down into the following three areas:

Maintenance
Electrical/mechanical engineering
Plumbing services
Note: There is a single maintenance contract for both sites

Hotel services
Catering
Domestic
Switchboard
Sewing/linen
Note: Hotel services include portering services at Stonehouse

Portering
Night security
Parking control
Transport services
Note: There is no separate portering contract for Stonehouse

Figures 12a and 12b illustrate the service contract arrangements for Hairmyres and Stonehouse hospitals.

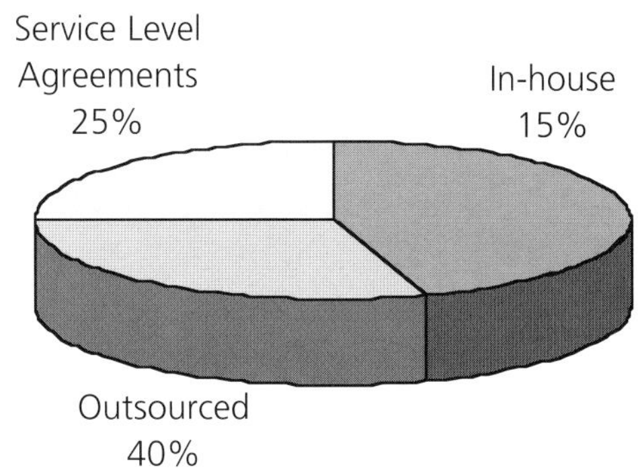

Figure 12a: Non-clinical services at Hairmyres

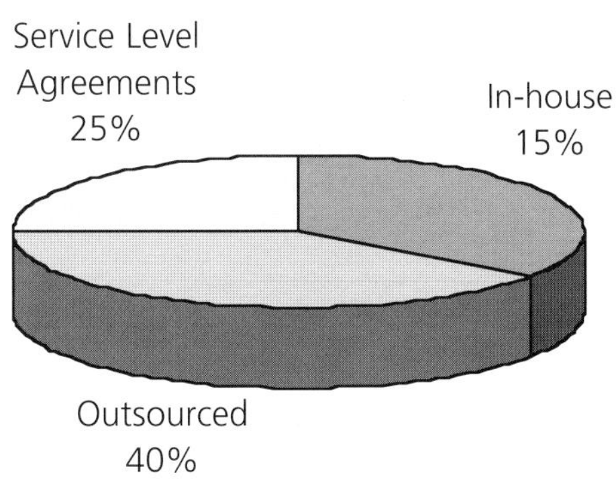

Figure 12b: Non-clinical services at Stonehouse

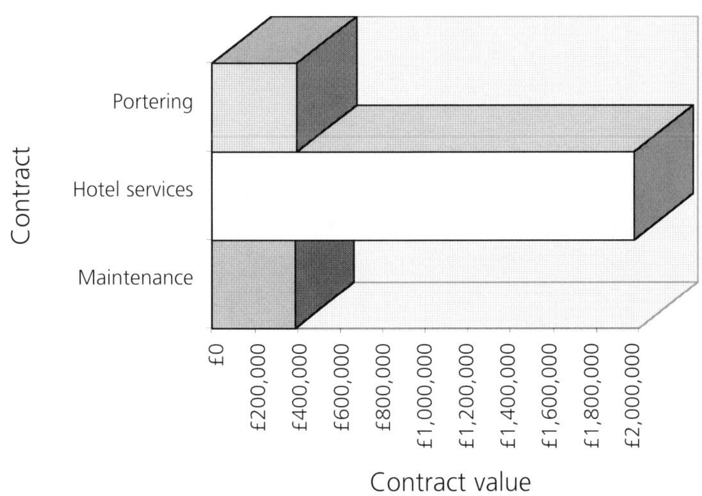

Figure 13: Total contract values

Contract values

The bar chart in Figure 13 shows the contract values for the three service groups. Hotel services account for the largest sum at just under £2m per annum.

Service contract staff

The distribution of staff under contract at the trust is illustrated in table 6.

Current contracts	Hairmyres	Stonehouse
Maintenance		
Electrical/mechanical Engineering Plumbing services Joiner services	21 *WTE for both sites	
Hotel services		
Catering Domestic Switchboard Sewing/linen	98 *WTE	43 *WTE
Portering		
Night security Parking control Transport services	35 *WTE	13 *WTE

*Whole Time Equivalent

Table 6: Number of staff under contract

Cost savings

Through the establishment and implementation of clear FM procedures, considerable cost savings are projected over the next five years in the area of non-clinical FM service provision. The greatest savings will be at Stonehouse Hospital where a predicted £227,000 is to be saved for the annual multi-services contract. At Hairmyres, annual savings in the region of £77,000 are expected to be made in the multi-services contract. Additional savings of £13,000 on the portering contract are also anticipated trust-wide. In total the trust hopes to save more than £1,769,000 in the next five years as each contract comes up for renewal.

These savings are a clear indication of the progress that can been made in a short time when the right strategies are put into place.

Future developments

PFI has provided an opportunity for the trust to procure a new hospital and thus improve the quality and efficiency of the healthcare environment. The trust has carried out a detailed clinical review of patient flows and functional relationships to produce a proposal for a state-of-the-art hospital which will meet the healthcare needs of its patients by the turn of the century.

As part of this process, detailed output specifications for all FM services have been prepared and agreed. Mechanisms for producing activity related costs, monitoring service performance, and imposing service failure penalties have also been determined. One area that was recognised as being significant to all of these plans was the impact that service failure could have on a building's availability. This point has been addressed fully between the trust and the consortium.

All FM services will be based on output specifications and will promote the use of generic workers. The generic team approach has been developed to maximise operational efficiency through multi-skilling at the margin of the traditional service boundaries. This merging of cultures aims to ensure that FM staff become fully integrated members of ward and departmental teams.

The trust's emerging FM culture concentrates on patient-focused care and fully adopts the quality, value and risk-led initiatives. It is hoped that this approach will result in a better healing environment and an improved working environment for a hospital of the future.

Analysis

The Hairmyres and Stonehouse hospitals case focuses on the evolution of facilities organisations through consolidation, rationalisation and restructuring. It deals with refocusing the service on patients and on developing a service culture and prioritising service objectives.

The case demonstrates a driving mission to link strategic objectives for the planning, provision and management of facilities to corporate objectives.

The issues that emerge from this case have an emphasis on management, and highlight the need for culture change and the development of the intelligent client function. Motivation, team building and communications are recurrent themes that reinforce the human dimension central to facilities management – people providing services to support people.

Milton Keynes General NHS trust

This case study examines how facilities management (FM) is helping Milton Keynes General NHS trust to meet its business objectives. The cornerstones of the trust's approach are quality, value and risk management. A comprehensive staff training programme is also seen as key to the creation of a successful FM culture.

Trust mission statement

'Milton Keynes General NHS trust aims to be a centre of excellence, recruiting, developing and retaining our staff to provide accessible, high quality, cost-effective local healthcare for our patients in an environment of education and research.'

The FM directorate bases its strategy and policy development on the principles of this statement.

Trust profile

Number of beds	475
Size of site	22 acres
Current value of estate	£51.0 million
Annual income	£41.0 million
Staff	1,318
Total floor area	48,516 m^2
FM directorate budget	£5.2 million

Background

Milton Keynes Hospital was initially commissioned in May 1984 to meet the local healthcare needs of Milton Keynes, a new town established in the 1970s and 1980s. The trust was created in April 1992 when the original hospital divided into two separate trusts – acute and community. The trust still provides many estate and facility services to the community trust.

Milton Keynes is a modern, purpose-built 457 bed hospital. The hospital initially provided 289 beds served by four operating theatres, with out-patient facilities mainly off site. The site was expanded in the 1980s to almost double its initial size with the commissioning in 1991 of an additional 168 beds and four operating theatres, together with a purpose built out-patients department. The trust is set in pleasant landscaped grounds of approximately 22 acres. The architecture is of modern design and was constructed using the "Oxford Method" developed by the old Oxford Regional Health Authority.

Corporate level

Development of facilities management services

The FM directorate was created at the inception of the trust and was formed from a mixture of estate and hotel service functions. The FM director was an experienced estates manager who took a pro-active role in the directorate's initial conception and subsequent development. The approach was to clearly identify strategic, tactical and operational functions. Individual areas of responsibility and accountability were clearly defined to foster an empowered environment.

Organisational structure

The FM director is one of five executive directors on the trust board. The organisational structure adopted in the FM directorate is shown in Figure 14.

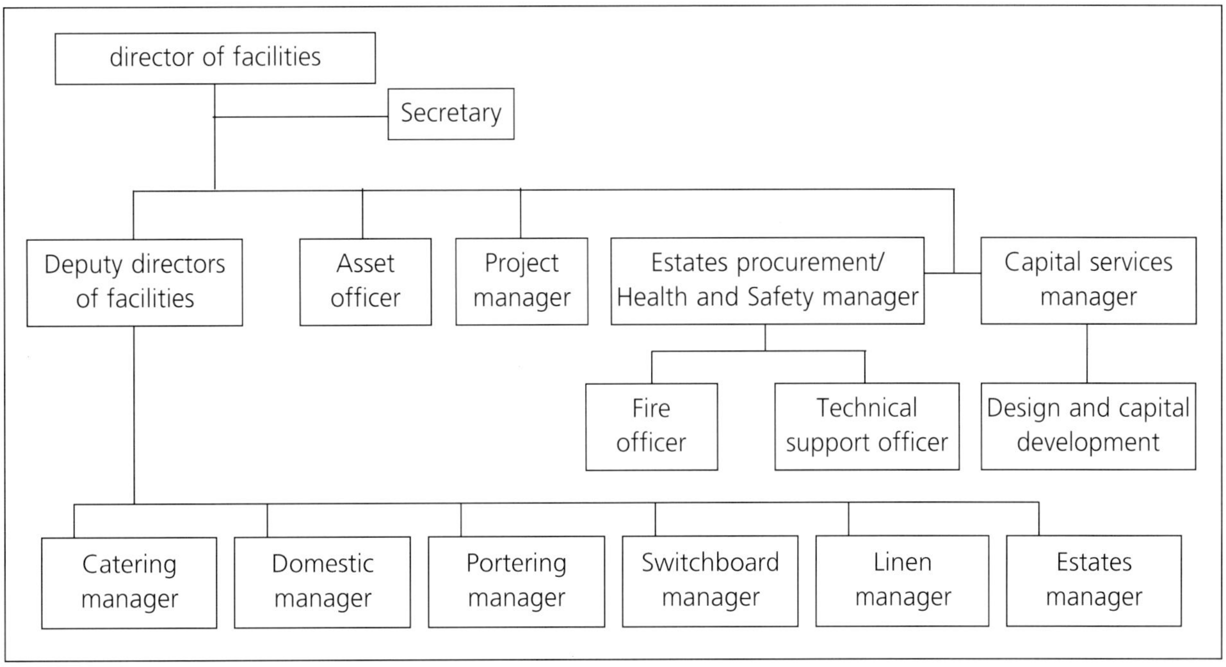

Figure 14: Facilities directorate structure

Strategic level

Strategic direction

The facilities strategy is:

> 'To provide a safe environment in which to deliver patient care. To maintain accommodation and support services to the standard required to facilitate and promote the trust activity with minimum risk to efficiency and personal safety and to be constantly prepared to change.'

The strategy applies to the following services which are managed by the directorate:

- Hotel services;
- Supplies service;
- Maintenance of the estate and assets;
- Transport – non-emergency ambulance services;
- Fire, security, waste disposal, energy and legislation relating to the environment;
- Capital development;

The FM director is also responsible for leading the trust's corporate risk management programme.

The FM directorate's budget is allocated in accordance with the pie chart shown in Figure 15.

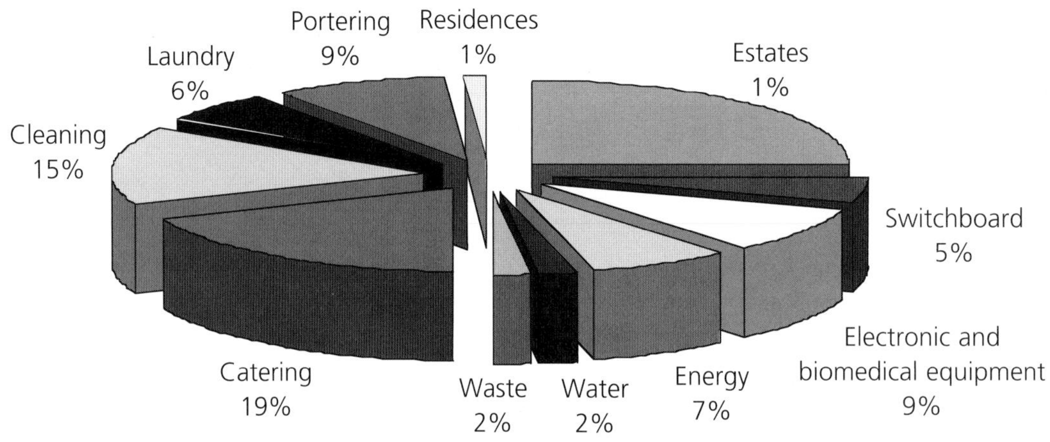

Figure 15: Facilities management expenditure 1995/96

Critical success factors

In moving gradually from a fragmented to an integrated organisation, the FM directorate has identified Critical Success Factors (CSFs) that will give maximum benefit in moving the trust forward. The business needs of the trust have been matched with financial and human resources to achieve a logical programme of change and implementation. The CSFs for the directorate are:

- to develop and introduce service level agreements;
- to develop all staff;
- to introduce and develop risk management;
- to develop a commercial value-for-money approach to all FM services;
- to develop performance management;
- to improve and develop communications.

Good communication with all involved has been a central issue in achieving the objectives. The aim is to create a site that is friendly, with a supportive atmosphere, for example Christian names are used at all levels.

Estate management

The trust has a sound understanding of its existing estate, and recognises the need for pro-active estate management. Functional suitability and space utilisation studies have been carried out to ensure the most economic use of space within the trust. The FM director is responsible for the allocation of space across the trust. To assist in this process, Computer Aided Facility Management (CAFM) software is currently being implemented to identify who occupies space in the trust.

The trust's estate management policy is broadly based on 'An exemplar estate strategy', published by NHS Estates. This approach ensures that government policy, purchasers' strategy and the trust's strategic direction are integrated and fully considered in the business planning process. The contribution that the estate can make to meeting the overall business strategy is recognised and valued at the trust, due in large part to the fact that the FM director is a member of the trust board.

The directorate is responsible for the delivery of the capital programme and the commissioning and monitoring of all professional services required.

The trust has an advantage over many other trusts in that all buildings have been constructed within the last 15 years to relatively recent standards. The trust does have backlog maintenance issues, however, many of which result from design weaknesses of the Oxford building method. The requirement to meet changing statutory and NHS current best practice also adds to this list.

Tactical level

Generic working

The trust has recognised that patients are becoming increasingly "service" sensitive. The NHS reforms, and the Patients' Charter in particular, have resulted in higher expectations, which in turn have fuelled the demand for a new approach to service delivery. The trust is planning to meet these expectations by the introduction of generic working.

As a starting point, generic working is being piloted on a six month basis at ward level. The approach taken has been to review the functional requirements at ward level and to examine how the various tasks are carried out. The central focus has been on customer care and quality. Value for money has been improved by transferring some duties, such as bed making, from qualified nursing staff to generic workers.

Generic working requires a multi-skilled approach and cuts across traditional job functions. Careful selection of staff is essential, they must be prepared to be flexible and develop their skill base. The pilot project attracted a high level of interest from both existing and new staff.

Successful generic working requires a change in attitude at all levels of the organisation. Staff must be empowered and motivated to carry out a wider range of tasks. The central features of the trust's approach to generic working are to:

- enhance the content of the work;
- expand the skills and tasks that make up the job;
- foster creativity and innovation;
- give staff greater control over decisions about work;
- enable staff to complete a whole task rather than merely portions of it;
- achieve customer satisfaction.

The training and development of staff was seen as key to the introduction of generic working. A comprehensive programme was developed, including specialist training in customer focus, quality, problem solving and team working. The overall aim was to extend each individual's skill range to meet customers' needs, while maintaining an optimum balance of skills across the range of generic workers.

Value for money

In the current economic climate, achieving value for money is a high priority for all service providers. The trust's FM directorate has either market tested or carried out a value analysis of the following services. The outcomes are shown in Table 7.

Non-clinical services	Contract
Linen services	In-house, with a contracted laundry service in a consortium of nine trusts
Cleaning	In-house
Portering	In-house
Catering	In-house (external cook chill contract)
Grounds	Outsourced
Non-emergency ambulance service	Outsourced
Car parking	In-house
Security	In-house
Window cleaning	Outsourced
Accommodation	Staff residences – all but two leased from housing association

Table 7: Contracts for non-clinical services

Service contracts are based on a mix of output and prescriptive specifications. The trust has aimed to achieve an appropriate blend of contracted and in-house services that balances quality, value and risk.

Risk management

Risk management has been recognised by the trust as one of the key areas for development over the next year. The FM director is responsible for developing the corporate risk strategy policy.

Service Level Agreements

Service Level Agreements (SLAs) have recently been introduced. They are designed to encourage the development of cost-effective services to meet business needs and to support the trust's objectives.

Historically, customers had little control over the cost or quality of services provided. Services were shaped by those providing them, and tended to be unresponsive to users' needs. SLAs have changed this culture by requiring service levels to be agreed between providers and users, and by making the service provider accountable to the customer.

The main benefits of SLAs are that they:

- align service to business needs;
- promote customer orientation;
- promote cost-effective service solutions;
- assist monitoring customer satisfaction;
- require management decisions on the appropriate quality and quantity of service.

SLAs require a commitment from service provider and customer, resources for their development, and they cannot improve a fundamentally poor service.

The trust's SLAs have sought to:

- reflect achievable targets;

- have tolerance for problems;
- define appropriate quality;
- be relevant;
- meet realistic customer expectations;
- seek consistency of response;
- detail remuneration arrangements;
- identify escalation arrangements.

Benchmarking

Benchmarking has been the cornerstone of establishing efficient and effective facility management functions.

The trust has adopted the Healthcare Facilities Consortium (HFC) benchmarking model. This has enabled critical analysis of the use and cost of space within the various directorates.

The FM directorate also carries out internal benchmarking and provides a quarterly report to the trust board on the performance – in terms of finance and customer service – of each directorate. This information is also presented to directorate managers in a monthly report. These reports have raised the profile of the directorate and provided sound information for strategic decision making.

Operational level

Security

The trust is improving security on the site and has made a commitment to comply with 'Preventing crime in the NHS'. The car park attendants' duties have been extended to provide 24 hour security across the hospital site.

Cycle routes from the hospital to Milton Keynes town centre are a potential security problem, as they provide access and egress routes for petty criminals. Specific measures have been taken to improve the security of the maternity unit.

The security strategy, together with other health and safety policies, will be progressively integrated into the trust's risk management strategy.

Future developments

Facilities management is well established at the Milton Keynes General NHS trust. It is playing a vital role in helping the trust to meet its business objectives and has provided a vehicle for change. The appointment of the FM director at board level has enabled the directorate to make a direct contribution to strategic decision making.

Analysis

Milton Keynes specific facilities mission is to provide a safe environment, maintain accommodation and support services, minimise risk and preparedness for change, explicitly related to the corporate business plan.

Milton Keynes identifies its critical success factors as meeting expectations, communication, attitude, training, flexibility, culture fit, and understanding the boundaries.

The basis and key role of effective facilities management in the delivery of healthcare is information. Milton Keynes reporting systems provide summary information on costs and performances which enable effective business planning. Benchmarking information is used to measure performance thus creating a balanced economy of contracted out and in-house services to balance quality, value and risk.

Northampton Community Healthcare NHS trust

Since its formation, Northampton Community Healthcare NHS trust has encountered a number of problems. Despite this, it is committed to improving the quality of its services and has adopted a FM approach to help achieve its aims. This case study looks at the way that FM services have been developed.

Trust mission statement

'To take health services to the people, only taking people to health services where absolutely necessary, whether their needs are physical, mental or disabling in nature.'

trust profile

Size of site	22 acres
Income 1995/96	£38 million derived from: Health authorities (38%) GP fundholders (4%) other sources (10%).
Current value of estate	£42 million
Total floor area	58,200 m^2
FM budget	£6.5 million (including capital charges)

Background

The Northampton Community Healthcare NHS trust was formed in April 1994. It provides primary care, learning disability and mental health services from 38 centres which include hospitals, GP practices, health centres and day hospital facilities. An associate director of facilities has recently been appointed.

Corporate level

Development of facilities management services

The newly-formed trust inherited a poorly maintained estate that did not match current or future business needs. Non-core business services were provided in a segmented fashion by a range of managers and the quality of service provision was poor. There was no clearly defined and co-ordinated strategy for meeting customers' expectations, and staff morale was low.

Capital charges have been a major financial problem for the trust, mainly as a result of the trust taking property into its portfolio that was not required for its business agenda. Many of these properties are surplus to requirements and can now be disposed of; however, the book value is far lower than the commercial sale value.

The trust had problems in three main areas:

- managing customers;
- managing services;
- managing assets.

Change was required to resolve the problems, and FM was chosen as the ideal vehicle to provide the innovation and framework by which change could be achieved.

The FM department was officially formed on 1 April 1996 from separate works and hotel services departments at three different management units.

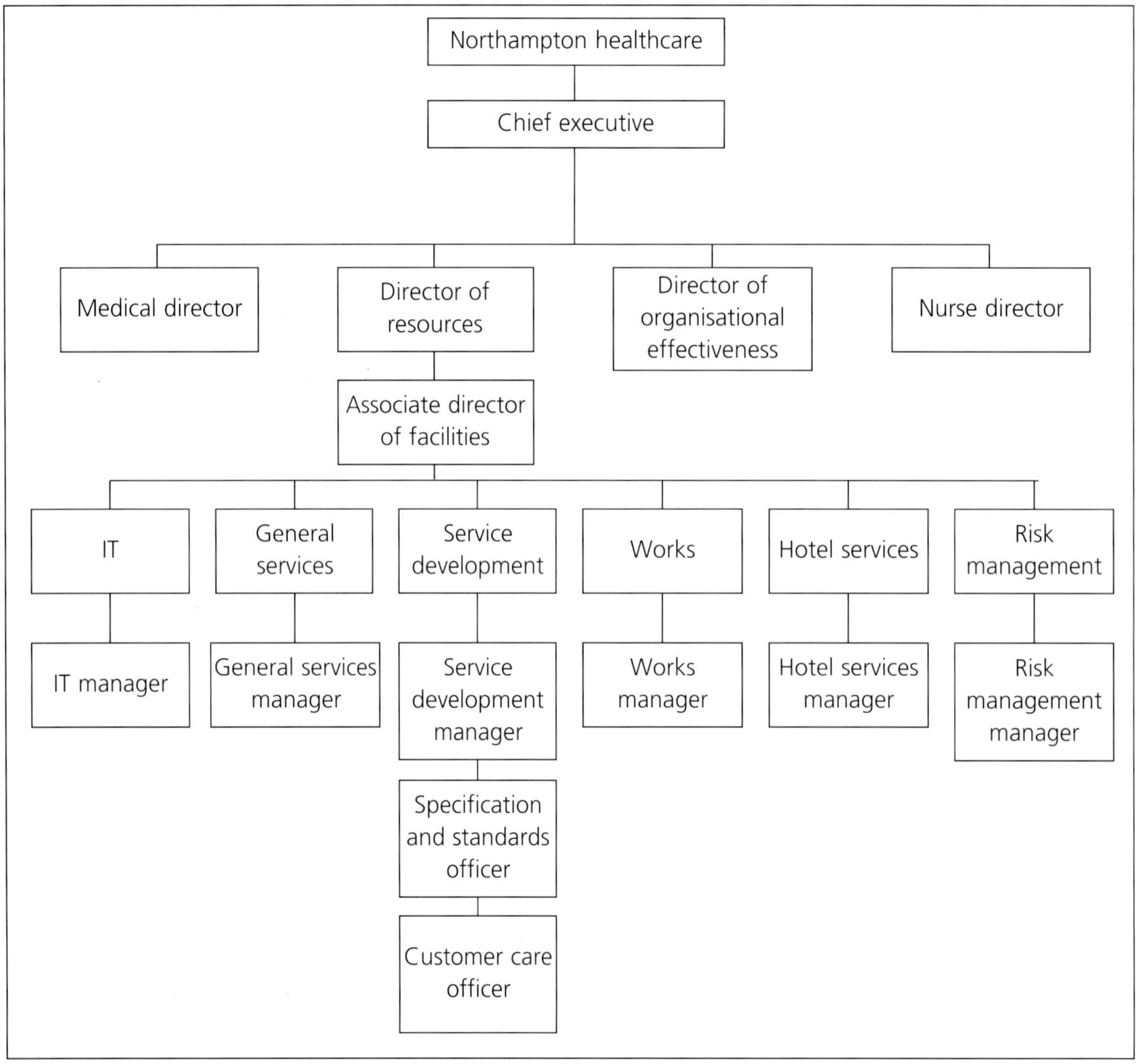

Figure 16: Facilities directorate structure

Facilities management mission statement

The department's philosophy is that:

> 'The services provided will be high quality, cost effective, responsive and focused on supporting the provision of patient care and the corporate objectives of the trust.'

The main objectives of the FM directorate were identified as follows:

- to provide a flexible estate capable of meeting changing business needs;
- to offer customer-focused services;
- to develop service level agreements, using a systematic service appraisal based on quality, value and risk;
- to ensure the holistic management of non-core services.

Quality, risk and value management are seen as the foundation stones of the FM directorate.

Strategic level

Strategic management

There are several factors which set the facilities business agenda, for example; trust objectives, finance, property requirements, risk, and probity. The FM strategy is seen as vital for the business agenda to be delivered. At Northampton, the FM strategy has been evolving in its first year through regular team meetings with senior staff where they are encouraged to question the way things are carried out. The approach is best described by the model of an inverted triangle with senior management supporting service delivery at the interface with the departments customers.

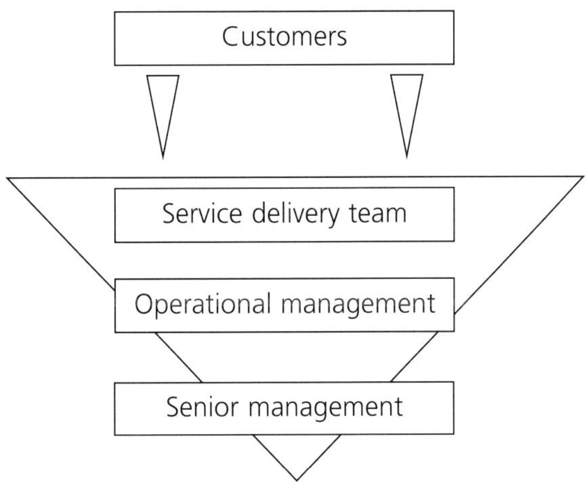

Figure 17: Management model

An organisation's strategy could be perceived as its personality. A strong, well developed FM strategy will give strength and stability to both the department and the trust. At Northampton, the emerging FM strategy is helping to earn the department a reputation for problem solving and good service delivery. This strength comes from a concentration on:

- people;
- skills;
- values;
- procedures;
- frameworks;
- culture.

The FM department's philosophy is that an empowered workforce which is able to take decisions and solve problems is the best way to deliver services. However, it is recognised that this method takes time to develop and effort is being put into both the people and the framework to assist this process. Future initiatives are to include training, possibly through the 'Investors in People' programme.

The new FM structure has defined areas of management, all of which combine to deliver the services required:

- general services;
- service development;
- works services;
- hotel services;
- risk management;
- information technology.

Each of these management units has well defined roles and responsibilities and is headed by a senior manager with appropriate support staff. These managers are developing a framework of support and guidance to allow staff to work effectively and make their own decisions in the workplace without fearing the consequences of "sticking their neck out".

More work is being done in this area of strategy development but indications to date are that staff welcome the change.

Estate management

An important element of the trust's strategy, as well as the FM strategy, is the management of its property portfolio. One of the early tasks of the associate director of facilities was to formulate an estate property strategy, which has now been completed and accepted by the trust board. A business case is being prepared to look at future options, which will involve re-profiling the property holding and examining the way in which that property is used.

At its inception, the trust inherited a number of properties that were only partly occupied. As a result, space utilisation of the buildings is poor. Although it is not easy for the trust to divest itself of surplus property, it has carried out a review to examine the possibility of reducing its estate. The report concluded that the trust will, over a period of time, be able to reduce the size of the estate by:

- restructuring the space usage in the town centre properties and selling off the larger buildings;
- transferring a number of services to the Mansfield Hospital site. This site is seen as community based and will enable the ultimate closure of the larger Princess Marina site;
- close down workshop and stores areas, replacing them with mobile units to suit the new working practices;
- the purchase of smaller properties and selling of larger properties to improve space utilisation.

To guide the rationalisation process, the trust has developed a set of principles:

- the trust estate should be "service" led not building led;
- wherever possible the trust should, with the exception of any future PFI partners, occupy buildings owned only by itself;
- the trust should retain only those buildings and lands that it requires for its own current or potential future use;

- a percentage of the trust's discretionary capital should be allocated annually to ensure the trust estate is well maintained. Buildings should be:
  - well placed;
  - of good quality;
  - well maintained;
  - secure;
  - energy efficient;
  - fit for purpose;
  - environmentally pleasing;
  - easily accessible to staff and users;
  - close to public transport;
  - utilised to their maximum.

The moves that are required will be complex and in some cases the temporary relocation of services will be necessary. The first phase has been approved by the trust board.

Tactical level

Teamworking

Teamworking and multi-skilling are seen as key to the successful delivery of facilities services. Generic working is being introduced in some areas, for example, maintenance staff are now trained and equipped to carry out a wide range of maintenance activities and are dedicated to a particular location or group of properties. This has achieved an improved standard of maintenance and staff appear to derive greater satisfaction from their work.

Over the next 12 months it is intended to develop generic working methods in areas of housekeeping such as cleaning, portering and catering by creating multi-skilled teams of staff who are integrated to meet the needs of a particular location. Discussion centres at present on the most appropriate number and size of teams. One element that has already been agreed is that there is insufficient synergy between works maintenance and housekeeping to justify combined teams. The size, number and location of each team will vary and therefore whilst being supportive of each other, the two functions will be managed separately at an operational level.

Risk management

The starting point for the trust has been the development of a risk management strategy which is supported and endorsed by the trust Board. Clinical and non-clinical risk management are identified as separate disciplines. Members of the risk management group include:

- Chief executive officer;
- Associate director of facilities;
- director of resources;
- director of nursing;
- Associate director of personnel;

- Control of infection officer;
- Risk manager (FM);
- Occupational health representative.

Each directorate is responsible for identifying its risks. Support and training opportunities are provided by the risk management department.

A risk assessment register has been developed to assist in the analysis process, at the same time giving a very good summary document of the trust's current position. This register is used to identify and summarise the risk control measures that are being implemented. As with most risk management strategies, insurance is used as the final back stop of control measures. The risk register to date has focused on the more obvious risks and how these are controlled and managed. More complex issues such as reputation risk and political risk will now be assessed and managed.

Risk management will be used as a vehicle for change, enabling the trust to comply with statutory requirements and develop a culture that is responsive to current and future pressures.

Value for money

An area of strategy identified for review is supply chain management. NHS Supplies currently carries out the major purchasing activity, although the service development manager has expressed concern as to whether real value for money is being achieved. If the trust is to meet its financial targets then a clear framework is needed to guide the day-to-day purchasing activity of its managers. This framework should address:

- cost;
- delivery schedules;
- quality;
- approved vendors/contractors;
- EU procurement rules;
- advantage from term contracts;
- tendering procedures;
- ethical and probity issues.

The devolvement of FM budgets to business units is seen as a possible way of introducing control and accountability. This has been tried in four properties within the town centre, but the outcome has been very disappointing, with overspent budgets, no control of standards and a degradation of the building stock. These budgets will be drawn back into FM control, and devolvement in the future will be undertaken on a service-by-service basis with FM providing a service framework and business units taking responsibility for controlling usage. For example, a centrally provided telephone service that is charged to business units according to usage.

Ensuring value for money is seen as key to the success of both FM and the trust. It is essential that value decisions are made by FM staff at all levels of the organisation. To enable this to happen a strong central framework is needed to guide staff and provide feedback regarding performance. At Northampton several developments are taking place to provide this framework, such as:

- marketing testing;
- benchmarking;
- performance management;

- service level agreements.

Future developments

In the first year since the introduction of FM at Northampton there appears to have been vast improvement in the quality of Northampton Community Healthcare trust's built environment and support services. The trust is now ready to build on this success and is about to start measuring its performance.

The culture has shifted towards empowered decision making and already a strong policy framework has been developed to guide the activities of staff at management, supervisory and operative levels. Further work will be carried out in this area as staff are encouraged to accept more responsibility for flexible and effective delivery. Multi-skilling and teamworking will be extended to the housekeeping functions throughout the coming year.

Risk management within the facilities department was built on previous health and safety policies and is now well developed with solid policies and procedures in place. The FM department is taking the leading role within the trust for all non-clinical risk management, which is used to set the agenda for capital development, strategic direction and service delivery. The trust's reputation is important to its future survival; reputation risk will therefore be an important issue and must be handled carefully as the trust endeavours to improve its standing within the local community and the NHS internal market.

The problems relating to the trust's high capital charge brought about by its inappropriate and overvalued property portfolio are being addressed. The principal solutions have been identified but work is now required to determine in more detail moves, disposals and acquisitions. The trust has recognised the need for professional estate and facilities advice at a strategic level.

A framework for achieving value and measuring performance is now being developed. Market testing of the three main services of cleaning, catering and laundry are being examined. Another initiative under consideration is the development of Service Level Agreements linked to the devolution of certain functional elements of the FM budget for example, cleaning, telephones, laundry.

The use of benchmarking as part of the trust's performance measurement programme is being considered. The business manager is examining the available services and is also trying to identify any benchmarking "clubs" managing similar community facilities.

The managers within the FM department are all committed to aiding and developing their staff by providing good training and strategic frameworks to allow the individuals and the organisation to flourish. By developing a risk management strategy, the trust is hoping to improve its property, services and image to deliver an appropriate level of service to the community it serves.

Analysis

This case study highlights the lead role that facilities managers are assuming in developing the corporate risk strategy. This strategy is normally built around the issues surrounding health and safety. At Northampton, risk management in seen as the change agent and the culture of the facilities directorate is being developed around the emerging strategy.

As with each of the cases, Northampton NHS trust recognises the importance of team building and multi-skilling and the need for training to enable staff to become responsive, flexible and innovative.

Worcestershire Community Healthcare NHS trust

This case study considers the challenges and benefits that have arisen from the merger of two small trusts into one organisation. The new trust is in the early stages of its development and the process is ongoing but a key element is the creation of an FM department.

Trust mission statement

'Milton Keynes General NHS trust aims to be a centre of excellence, recruiting, developing and retaining our staff to provide accessible, high quality, cost-effective local healthcare for our patients in an environment of education and research.'

'To provide, develop and lead effective healthcare in our community.'

The aims of the trust are to:

- support patients and carers in the community by grouping services around GPs;
- provide high quality/cost effective services through well trained staff;
- enable patients to have a choice about treatment and care;
- stimulate research and to lead the development of new/best clinical practice;
- be a good employer;
- be competitive.

Trust profile

Number of beds	322
Number of staff	1,624 whole time equivalent
Annual income:	£44 million
Total assets:	£46 million
Property portfolio:	four community hospitals five mental health buildings 28 health centres and clinics 12 learning disabilities homes seven miscellaneous properties
Total floor area:	49,000 m^2
FM budget:	£7.2 million

Background

On 1 April 1996 the North East Worcestershire Community Healthcare trust and the South Worcestershire Community NHS trust were dissolved and replaced by the Worcestershire Community Healthcare NHS trust. The new trust sees the following as the main advantages of the merger:

- improved opportunities for service development;
- improved organisational resources to enable a more flexible approach for service planning and delivery;
- financial savings from merging that can be re-invested in patient care;

- long-term financial stability;
- the ability to respond to opportunities arising from the new mental health purchasing strategy for the county.

Corporate level

Development of facilities management services

Bringing together the two trusts has not been without difficulties as old loyalties and differing visions for the future exist. The new trust has continued to run the estate and services on traditional lines, but an FM structure has been formulated to include a senior facilities manager with overall responsibility.

The estates departments have had very different structures. The department in the northern section of the trust has a heavy management structure and highly developed procedures to produce detailed strategic information on property issues. However, responsiveness to service requests is seen to be poor and customer care in general could be improved. The emerging FM structure has been formulated specifically to deal with this issue.

The department in the south of the trust is focused on service delivery at ward and departmental level but still has a traditional task-oriented framework. Strategic advice is given by the acute trust under an inter-service agreement. Estates information is produced in a variety of ways. The Works Information Management System (WIMS) is used in the north of the trust for operational information, although no computer assisted information system exists for production of strategic information regarding the trust's property portfolio. This needs to be evaluated and a suitable system selected.

Hotel services are managed differently in the north and south of the trust. Although the estates manager has been re-titled 'facilities manager' in the south of the trust, hotel services throughout the trust operate independently of the estates function. There has been some market testing activity and domestic services are now provided by external contract in the south and by in-house contract in the north. Catering is largely provided by cook-chill, with prepared food provided by external contract and by inter-service agreement with a local acute trust.

The trust has analysed all functions currently carried out by estates and hotel services and has defined those which will now be managed by the new facilities department:

- estates strategy;
- estates operations;
- service planning;
- capital projects;
- electronic and biomedical equipment;
- risk (facilities related);
- domestic/housekeeping services;
- linen services;
- catering;
- grounds and gardens;
- portering and security;

- transport;
- telephone services.

It has been decided that trust information technology (excluding FM) should be managed by the business support director and where estates currently manage this activity a controlled handover will take place.

FM organisational structure

The trust has recognised that it can increase its competitive advantage by co-ordinating the management of its estate and facilities, and a new FM structure – based on teamworking – is being implemented. A facilities manager, reporting to the patient care director (who is a member of the trust board), will be appointed to manage the reorganisation. The central plank of the new structure will be the formation of three self-managing service delivery teams, each led by a service co-ordinator. Each team will have its own multi-skilled workers, recruited and trained to suit the needs of each particular locality. The co-ordinator will be directly accountable to the facilities manager, and will construct and agree patterns of work and programmes in conjunction with the locality manager to suit local requirements. The new structure is shown in Figure 18.

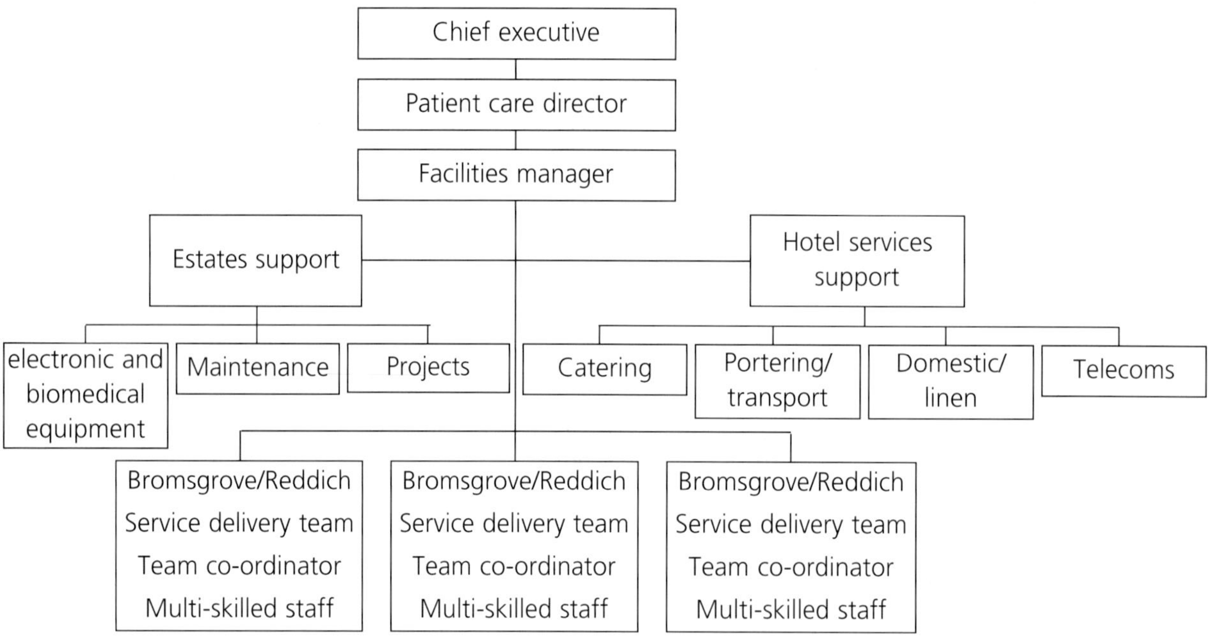

Figure 18: Facilities directorate structure

The service delivery teams will be supported by two specialist advisory teams, one providing estates support, the other providing hotel services support. These two teams will not have a line management responsibility but will exist to support service delivery by providing a wide range of services at operational and strategic level. The operational service elements will, however, always be co-ordinated by the local service delivery co-ordinator. The advisory teams will provide support by:

- setting up the necessary service and supply contracts;
- acting as internal contractor where it is better to retain skills in a specialist central team such as electronic and biomedical equipment maintenance;
- undertaking project work;
- carrying out market testing by tendering on a trust-wide basis;

- establishing standards;
- providing training and working to reduce risk to acceptable levels.

The teams will provide strategic advice on estate appraisal, for example, to assist the facilities manager in decision making.

Careful selection of the team co-ordinators will be required to ensure that they have the talents required to build a team that can meet the needs of the service user and operate within a mutually supportive framework. They will need to identify suitable training programmes that will extend competency levels within the team to match the particular skill levels required.

FM budget

The total cost of the new FM services represents 14% of total trust income (see Table 8). This figure is felt to be high and comparison of occupancy and support costs against Health Facilities Consortium (HFC) benchmarking data would support this view (see Table 9).

FM budget breakdown

Item	North	South	Total
Estates			
Managment	248,438	45,077	
Maintenance	289,390	454,116	
Equipment (non recuring)	20,000		
Office services	19,111		
Rates/general expenses	416,878		
Technical services	42,945		
Energy and utilities	286,038	245,539	
Hotel services			
Administration	40,215	26,322	
Catering	424,518	3,766,801	
External contracts	5,208	8,705	
Housekeeping	410,266	308,679	
Laundry	190,828	26,493	
Portering	52,051	141,417	
Telephones	16,453	0	
Training	10,494	0	
Transport	37,261		
Total	**2,889,074**	**1,6331,49**	**4,522,223**
Capital charges			**2,710,938**
Grand total			**7,233,161**
Trust income			**4,400,000**

Table 8: FM budget breakdown.

Occupancy cost

Item	North	South
Variable		
Management	249,438	45,077
Maintenance	289,390	315,259
Equipment (non recuring)	20,000	
Office services	19,111	
Tech services	42,945	
Information	42,622	
Energy and utilities	286,038	245,539
Housekeeeping	410,266	308,679
External contracts	5,208	8,705
Waste disposal	59,000	
Annual cost	1,424,018	923,259
Gross internal area	23,957	25,000
Cost per m²	59.00	37.00
Fixed		
Rates	308,878	138,857
Capital charges	2,710,938	1,576,062
Insurance	49,000	-
Annual cost	3068,816	1,714,919
Gross internal area	23,957	25,000
Cost per m²	128.00	69.00
Support		
Admin	40,215	26,322
Catering	424,518	376,801
Laundry	190,828	26,493
Portering	52,051	141,417
Annual cost	707,612	571,033
Gross internal area	23,957	25,000
Cost per m²	30.00	23.00

Trust totals	Per annum	Per m²
Variable	2,347,277	48.00
Fixed	4,783,735	98.00
Support	1,278,645	26.00
Gross internal area	48,957	
Occupancy cost		146.00

Table 9: Occupancy cost

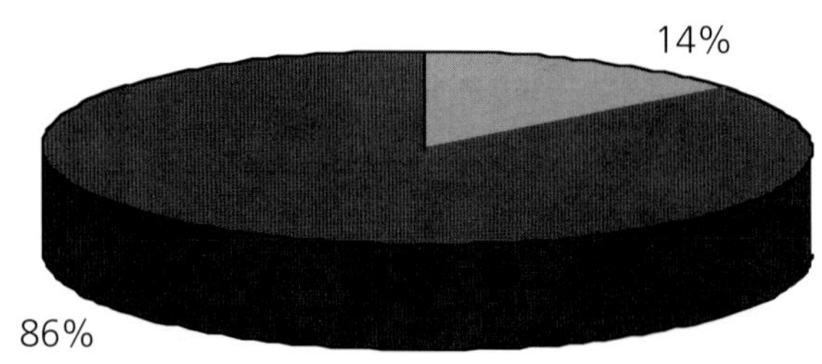

Figure 25: FM costs as % of trust income

The trust has defined savings targets and occupancy costs are seen as a significant contributor to these savings. Costing information is produced in two totally different styles and this needs to be rationalised to simplify analysis and reporting procedures. The calculation in Table 9 of fixed, variable and support costs is fairly "broad brush" but can be considered accurate enough for initial analysis. Using the HFC benchmarking data the occupancy cost (fixed + variable) appears to be high. The trust is looking for savings of £400,000 per annum for re-investment in patient care, with £150,000 of this sum coming from the facilities operation. This will involve a reduction in its fully serviced cost (fixed + variable + support) of £3 per square metre and comparison to the benchmarking data indicates that this is achievable. The fixed cost gives the widest variation, however, this can be difficult to reduce and the variable costs will be examined to achieve reductions in the short term to deliver the savings required by the trust.

Strategic level

Strategic direction

There are several priorities that will shape the introduction of FM but the four main areas for immediate action are:

- development of a facilities culture;
- formation of the service delivery teams;
- development of the advisory functions;
- development of an estates strategy.

To facilitate the change of culture which will be required to bring the separate estates and hotel services together under one FM umbrella, some workshops have been held, with a generally enthusiastic response from staff.

Estates strategy

An estates strategy will be developed to optimise the management of the trust's properties to meet its service and business needs. The bringing together of two property portfolios makes this a high priority for action. The strategy will cover:

- appraisal of the existing estate;
- proposed changes;
- estate control plan;
- estate rationalisation programme;
- investment programme;
- acquisitions and disposal programme.

The methodology described in 'An exemplar estates strategy', published by NHS Estates, will be used as the framework for the study. An efficient facilities information system and some modest investment will be necessary.

Tactical level

Quality

Although the trust has not yet formulated its policy for the achievement of quality, it is committed to providing quality patient-focused healthcare services to the community it serves. It is recognised that the environment and "front of house" services create the first impressions that can influence patients' and visitors' perceptions of the quality of the overall service provided by the hospital. The facilities department pays careful attention to quality in these areas.

To ensure that facilities are of the highest quality and appropriate to the specific task the north section of the trust has developed a database detailing condition, compliance with statutory standards, space utilisation and functional suitability. At present the south section buys this service in from the local acute trust on an inter-service agreement. This information will be rationalised into one co-ordinated document which will take account of the new trust's objectives and cover all properties to ensure that the built environments are appropriate.

The trust recognises the importance of effective management, maintenance and development of its estate to meet changing service needs. Most of the buildings in the north of the trust are new and it is not envisaged that any large capital investment will be necessary in the foreseeable future. The emphasis will lie in ensuring that the buildings are accessible to all and that it provides a safe and pleasant environment. The south of the trust has few modern buildings although considerable repair and renewal has been carried out in the recent past. Within the last three years extensions to the estate at the Evesham, Malvern and Worcester City sites have taken place. Considerable progress has been made with the provision of access for the disabled.

The primary responsibility for quality in the provision of FM services will fall on the self-managing teams. This approach will encourage :

- teams that are pro-active rather than re-active;
- a "one stop" style providing quicker responses for service users;
- a problem solving approach to enable the total care process;
- an empowered framework responsive to the needs of service users.

Teamworking

A multi-skilled approach is to be applied to enable flexible services to develop. Breaking the mould of rigid organisational structures, each team will take ownership of a specified locality and will possess an appropriate level of skills. Individuals within the team will be trained in order to widen their personal scope and enable them to perform as generic workers. The traditional boundaries between skilled and non-skilled workers will not necessarily be abandoned, but they are being blurred to gain maximum benefit from the available staff. Team members will be encouraged to develop their personal range of skills to maximise their potential and to contribute to the wide variety of jobs the team is required to perform.

Careful selection of the team co-ordinators and the correct balance of skills within a team are seen as keys to success. Whilst generic working will be a feature of the new work style the emphasis will be on flexibility and teamworking in a supportive framework. In the interest of safety some skill boundaries will be retained. For example, it would not be economic to train all staff in food hygiene when some staff would never carry out those duties. However, by accepting that some duties can, with suitable training, be safely carried out by several different staff groups, overall team performance can be enhanced. Service is seen as a matrix of tasks, skills and people which, if combined effectively, can deliver significant improvements in service quality.

The role of the advisory teams will need to be defined; the shift from line manager to that of internal consultant or contractor will be a major cultural change for those involved. Training, consultation and, ultimately, acceptance of this new style of working may not be easy to achieve. Their role will be to enable the delivery of facilities service at both strategic and operational levels by giving good professional leadership.

Value management

It is the trust's aim to achieve value for money in the provision of FM services. It strongly subscribes to the view that value is the achievement of necessary function for minimum cost whilst achieving quality, reliability and good performance.

It is seen as essential that high quality information is available to enable the facilities manager to quantify value and measure performance. The FM database will be reviewed and managed by the estates advisor to ensure that the correct information to assist strategic and operational decision making is available. The key to providing value is the ability to react flexibly to changing needs and the facilities information system must be able to show accurately for each asset its fixed and variable costs. The system will be developed to ensure this is achievable.

Measurement and comparison are important features of a value management system and this will be achieved through performance management and benchmarking.

The hotel services advisor will lead the collation of information for benchmark comparison through one of the recognised healthcare benchmarking services. This information will be used for annual reviews of overall performance as well as for focused studies and reports on specific aspects of the service. Performance measurements will be developed to complement the benchmarking activity and regular reports will be made to the board regarding the value of FM activity. It is felt that, in keeping with the trust's general philosophy that the patient/client is central to service delivery, it is essential that the less tangible aspects of FM services, such as general client satisfaction and perceived response time etc., are assessed. To achieve this regular surveys will be undertaken of the service users. The results will be tabulated and quantified and linked to appropriate action plans, which will be published and re-measured at regular intervals. The process will apply equally to contracted and in-house services.

Risk strategy

The trust is building a risk strategy which is based on the best practice from each of the former trusts. The business support director has overall responsibility and has formed a risk management group that he sees as providing the framework to encourage innovation. Clinical and non-clinical risks are perceived as being inter-related parts of the overall risk management process, with each impacting on the other. The philosophy is that some risk associated with clinical activity will be reduced if that activity is carried out in well constructed and maintained buildings which are serviced at an appropriate level.

Insurance is being re-tendered for the new trust with the assistance of NHS Supplies and initially high premiums are expected. As the risk management group develops procedures, policies and safe systems of work, premiums are expected to reduce.

A number of good policies have already been formulated, for example, a "lone worker" policy (which is of particular relevance to a community trust) has been introduced, which gives advice and instruction on the following:

- responsibilities of employer and employee;
- late working;

- general safety precautions;
- the need to be accompanied on certain visits;
- use of mobile phones for security;
- action for vehicle breakdowns;
- community settings;
- potential violence;
- how to avoid hazardous situations.

The strategy takes account of 'Risk management in the NHS' and wherever possible will be developed from pre-existing good practice rather than re-invented. The Facilities Manager carries a major responsibility to understand, assess and translate into action the requirements of all legislation, codes of practice, and health and safety documentation relating to the built environment. The emphasis is on working to find solutions in a positive and pro-active manner rather than purely the identification of hazards.

The analysis of near miss situations as well as actual incidents is considered important in identifying potential risk. For example a recent near miss incident in an out-patient clinic showed that it was possible for a child to insert his hand into a sharps box through the lid. Fortunately no injury occurred but as a result the trust has analysed and tightened its procedures for the use of sharps containers. The ARRAN (Accident Recording, Reporting and Analysis System) has recently been introduced. This is a Windows-based system and early indications are that it is simple to use and the statistical analysis and reporting features are good.

A risk auditing tool has been developed by the former South trust which covers some 35 different topics. The methodology generally follows the NHS Manual framework with risk being classified as low, medium, significant or high. These assessments are then quantified and ranked and linked to a corrective action plan. The system will be extended and used throughout the trust.

Operational level

Staff training

An extensive programme of training is taking place throughout the trust at two levels:

a. senior manager; and

b. general staff.

Senior management training, which will include the facilities manager, has begun, with frequent workshops to introduce new ideas and promote two-way communication. A more formal programme is being developed in conjunction with Manchester University to include training in:

- leadership;
- teamworking;
- motivation;
- business planning;
- general management skills.

General staff training courses will be carried out internally by the human resources department, where sufficient skills already exist, with help co-opted from specialist managers where required. Programmes will be tailored to suit individual group needs and the facilities manager will work with the training team to ensure an effective programme for facilities staff at all levels.

Future developments

Worcestershire Community Healthcare NHS trust recognises that the FM function can significantly impact on the experience of individual patients by the quality of its built environments and the manner of delivery of its support services. The new facilities manager will formulate a precise mission for FM but the trust already perceives the priority to be providing quality buildings and appropriate support services to enable the delivery of high quality healthcare to the community.

The programme of change implies a major upheaval for all staff and the trust is anxious to allay any fears. The facilities manager will involve staff organisations at an early stage to establish a good working relationship.

It is fortunate that the formation of the facilities department is taking place in parallel with the formation of the trust. This is recognised as an opportunity to develop a service that is consistent with the overall aims and objectives of the organisation for the delivery of responsive healthcare services to the community.

Analysis

Worcestershire Community Healthcare NHS trust has enabled the evolution of facilities management through consolidation, rationalisation and restructuring. Refocusing the service on patients, developing a service culture and prioritising service objectives have all contributed to organisational development.

This has highlighted the need for effective team working and training, supported by a change in culture and development of the intelligent client function. Motivation, team building and communications are recurrent themes that reinforce the human dimension central to facilities management – people providing services to support people.

4.0 Conclusion

The selected case studies represent different stages in the development of FM in the NHS. In some cases, the trust is in the early throes of introducing an FM approach, in others it is relatively mature. At each stage there are fresh issues, new challenges and opportunities in the continuing process of adapting facilities to healthcare needs.

Each case demonstrates a driving mission to link FM strategic objectives to corporate objectives. There is a common belief that it is possible to enhance the organisation's effectiveness, build a positive image and create a more productive workplace through improving the quality of buildings and services. In some cases this is part of a vision, in others the ambitions are already beginning to be fulfilled.

The cases focus on the evolution of facilities organisations through consolidation, rationalisation and restructuring. They each deal with refocusing the service on patients, on developing a service culture and prioritising service objectives. They adopt different change agents – initiatives to improve quality, value and risk – through empowering a leaner internal team or through outsourcing. All the cases highlight the need for training in the "learning organisation".

Four key themes have emerged from the study:

- the need for effective corporate management;
- the importance of the role of the intelligent client;
- the need for continual process improvement;
- the need for organisational development.

Corporate management

The manner in which a trust is governed will determine the opportunities for effective FM. This must start with the commitment of the chief executive or chairman of the trust and their recognition that FM contributes to meeting healthcare objectives and business targets.

If FM is to be effective it must be planned as part of the trust's overall business strategy, which implies that facilities managers must either be members of the trust board or report directly to it. The Milton Keynes case study demonstrates how an innovative and dynamic facilities director at board level can introduce broad change across and beyond the traditional organisational boundaries.

The intelligent client

The most effective intelligent clients are those that can operate at two very different levels. They must have an overview of the FM service which enables them to see ahead, formulate policy and help define the trust's vision for the future. In addition, they must be in tune with the individuals who use the service, understanding what they need and how that demand may change in the future.

Continual process improvement

The case studies highlight the need to continually improve the management and delivery of facilities services. Many trusts are adopting the quality, value and risk management approach (described in Chapter 2) as a framework for assessing existing arrangements and identifying areas for improvement.

Ensuring high-quality services is now a prime objective for FM departments. One way of assessing quality is to measure customer satisfaction through, for example, surveys, quality audits, action groups, feedback mechanisms, and empowered involvement. At Hairmyres and Stonehouse NHS trust, which has been accredited by the Kings Fund, the number of complaints is used as a quality indicator. In fact, many trusts are underpinning their commitment to quality by accreditation against recognised standards such as ISO 9002, Investors in People, and the government-sponsored Charter Mark. Tools such as the Estates Quality Model and the 'An exemplar estates strategy' can provide a framework for improving the quality of estates management.

Allied with quality is the need to ensure that services are as cost effective as possible. Faced with increasing pressure to drive down costs, it is important to demonstrate that costs are related to overall performance. In other words, FM services must be seen to be contributing to the trust's overall business objectives. Benchmarking is becoming increasingly popular as a way of measuring the value, and to a lesser extent the quality, of facilities services. Benchmarking clubs provide members with a set of key indicators that are important in determining facilities performance. However, the definitions of such indicators should be standardised if comparisons are to be made on a like-for-like basis.

The management of risk is an essential task, and in many trusts it may fall to the facilities manager to take the lead in developing a corporate risk strategy. Identifying the risks to which a trust is exposed can provide a framework for developing and improving services, particularly in areas such as security, waste disposal, and health and safety. At Northampton NHS trust risk management is seen as a vehicle for change and the culture of the FM department is being shaped by the emerging risk strategy. The 'An exemplar risk management strategy' provides practical guidance on developing and implementing a risk management strategy.

Organisational development

trusts are dynamic and subject to changes in their environment: changes in legislation, working practices, and the development of new technologies, for example, can have an impact on day-to-day operations. Adapting to such change is vital to a trust's success and survival.

Facilities managers must develop approaches that enable positive change, whilst recognising that change can destabilise the organisation. Developing new working practices is one – often very difficult – aspect of changing the organisational culture to better fit business needs. Team building and multi-skilling, for example, can lead to a more responsive, flexible and innovative workforce but such changes must be supported by appropriate training and development schemes to ensure that staff acquire the necessary new skills. Creating an environment in which staff feel more empowered requires cultural change.

Conclusion

The aim of facilities management is to ensure that non-clinical services are high-quality, cost effective and contribute to the business needs of the trust. Central to this objective is the need for accurate information on facilities performance and direction in the form of a strategy linked to the trust's business plan. This should be supported by a staff development plan which encourages empowerment and innovation.

The unison of all these elements is the key to successful facilities management. Unfortunately such fundamental change is unlikely to take place overnight – it may take a trust months or even years to create a new environment – but the ultimate reward is continually improving services, satisfied customers and success for the facilities team.

5.0 Summary of good practice

Corporate

- Establishing a single FM directorate with responsibility for all non-clinical services will reduce overheads and help to ensure seamless services.
- There will be benefits to the organisation as a whole if the FM director has representation at board level and reports directly to the chief executive.
- A service-oriented culture should be developed.

Strategic

- The FM strategic plan should be consistent with the trust's business objectives. Underpinning the FM strategy with a mission statement can help to remind FM staff of their important role within the trust.
- An IT strategy should be developed to ensure that accurate and relevant data is captured and collated for reporting as required.
- There are advantages to be gained in appointing an "intelligent client" to act as a single point of contact for customers.
- A comprehensive marketing strategy should be developed based on the results of service audits and customer feedback.

Tactical

- Services should be continually monitored for quality and value. This is best achieved by identifying a range of "indicators" against which performance can be measured. The performance indicators should be closely linked to critical success factors.
- Sharing information with other trusts – through benchmarking clubs – can help a trust to improve its competitive advantage.
- The FM director is often well placed to take a lead role in developing a trust-wide risk management strategy.
- There are benefits to be gained from introducing more flexible working patterns, for example multi-skilling and generic workers.

Operational

- Staff training and development schemes should be tailored to meet the needs and priorities of the trust.
- Performance indicators should be monitored on a day-to-day basis.

Appendix I: Self-assessment checklist

This checklist provides a framework for trusts to carry out an initial assessment of their FM services.

Corporate objectives
How might the organisation's values and long-term goals affect the approach to FM?

Business planning
How might future changes in the healthcare market impact on FM provision?

Corporate culture
How important is teamwork to the trust?

Quality
Does the trust have an explicit quality policy outlining the following:

- high level of customer satisfaction;
- information management systems;
- feedback mechanisms providing data on satisfaction, response times and service continuity;
- accessibility and transparency of the process;
- staff development and training;
- space utilisation and service take up?

Value
Does the trust have a value action plan that:

- compares value management procedures and costs with other trusts;
- relates each cost centre to its objectives of enhancing asset value and delivering a cost-effective service;
- assesses whether value is being achieved at each stage of the process;
- reorganises the facilities to provide for continual improvement (culture change);
- manages revenue generation;
- provides a value management auditing process?

Risk
Does the trust have a risk management plan that considers:

- risk of loss to business;
- risk to human life or limb (that is, health and safety);
- risk of environmental failure;
- risk to the environment (pollution);
- risk to property;
- risk of physical failure;
- risk of financial loss and viability?
- Does the trust have established procedures for identifying, assessing and managing risk?
- Does the trust provide a risk management training/awareness programme for staff?

References

Akhlaghi, F. and Mahony, L. **Service integration and multi-skilling in facilities management within the UK National Health Service.** Facilities, 1997, vol 15, no 3/4, March/April.

BS EN ISO 9000: Quality management and quality assurance standards.

BS EN ISO 9002: 1994 Quality systems. Model for quality assurance in production, installation and servicing. BSI Standards.

BS 7750: 1994 Specification for environmental management systems. BSI Standards.

Capital Investment Manual

Overview. NHS Executive, The Stationery Office 1994.

Project organisation. NHS Executive, The Stationery Office 1994.

Private finance guide. NHS Executive, The Stationery Office 1994.

Business case guide. NHS Executive, The Stationery Office 1994.

Management of construction projects. NHS Estates, The Stationery Office 1994.

Commissioning of a healthcare facility. NHS Executive, The Stationery Office 1994.

IM&T Guidance. NHS Executive, The Stationery Office 1994.

Post project evaluation. NHS Executive, The Stationery Office 1994.

Clinical waste incineration – joint venture arrangement (Health Guidance Note). NHS Estates, The Stationery Office 1994.

Cordery, J.L. **Multi-skilling; a discussion of proposed benefits of new approaches to labour flexibility.** Personnel Review, 1989, March.

Estatecode

Volume 1: Strategic asset management

Estate investment planning

Analysis of estate performance

Asset maintenance. NHS Estates, The Stationery Office 1993.

Volume 2: Property transactions – a management guide for NHS trusts. NHS Estates, The Stationery Office 1994.

An exemplar estate strategy. NHS Estates The Stationery Office 1996.

An exemplar risk management strategy. NHS Estates, The Stationery Office 1997.

Facilities management measurement protocol. British Institute of Facilities Management (BIFM), 1995.

Firecode: policy and principles. NHS Estates, The Stationery Office 1994.

Firecode: fire risk assessment in nucleus hospitals. NHS Estates, The Stationery Office 1997.

Greencode. NHS in Scotland Healthcare Engineering and Environment Unit 1997.

Healthcare waste management – segregation of waste streams in clinical area (Health Technical Memoranda 2065). NHS Estates, The Stationery Office 1997.

Houston, A and McFadzean, E. **Study of facilities management practice in the UK 1994/95, Part 1: Facilities management practice in the NHS.** Centre for Facilities Management, University of Strathclyde, 1995.

Management of health and safety at work: Management of Health and Safety at Work Regulations 1992: approved code of practice. Health and Safety Commission, HSE Books 1992.

The New NHS (Cm 3808). The Stationery Office 1997.

Organisational audit (accreditation UK): standards for an acute hospital. 2nd ed. King's Fund Centre Quality Improvement Programme, King's Fund Centre 1990.

Organisational audit (accreditation UK): standards for an acute hospital. 2nd ed. King's Fund Centre Quality Improvement Programme, King's Fund Centre 1990.

Oxford method. Oxford Regional Hospital Board, 1971. (out of print)

The Patient's Charter. Department of Health, 1991.

The Patient's Charter and you. Department of Health, 1995.

Preventing crime in the NHS the management challenge: a review of security and crime prevention in the NHS. Crime Prevention Consulting, Department of Health 1993.

Re-engineering the facilities management service (Health Facilities Note 16). NHS Estates, The Stationery Office 1996.

Rees, D. **The current state of facilities management in the UK NHS: an overview of management structures.** Facilities, 1997, vol 15, no 3/4, March/April.

Risk management in the NHS. Merrett Health Risk Management Ltd. and NHS Management Executive, Department of Health, 1993.

Safe disposal of clinical waste – whole hospital policy guidance (Health Guidance Note). NHS Estates, The Stationery Office 1995.

A strategic guide to clinical waste management. NHS Estates, 1994.

Structure of the facilities management industry – Facilities management industry analysis: Issue 2. Centre for Facilities Management, University of Strathclyde, 1996.

Successful health and safety management (HS(G)65). Health and Safety Executive, HSE Books 1991.

Waste management the duty of care: a code of practice. Department of the Environment, 1996.

Webber, Chris. **Contracting for competitive NHS support services.** Harlow Longman, 1994.

Woodcock, M. and Francis, D. **Organisational development through teambuilding.** Gower, 1990.

Bibliography

Argyris, C. and Schon, D.A. **Organisational learning; a theory of action perspective.** Addison-Wesley, 1978.

Corporate governance in the NHS: Controls assurance statements (HSG(97)17). NHS Executive, Department of Health 1997.

Cotts, David. **The cost of ownership. Proceedings of Facilities Management International Conference, Glasgow 1990.** Centre for Facilities Management.

Cutler, B. **Getting ahead in slippers.** American Demographics, 1990, Feb, p11.

Ellram, Lisa. **Total cost of ownership: elements and implementation.** International Journal of Purchasing and Materials Management, 1993, Fall, p3-11.

Ferry, D.J.O. and Flanagan, R. **Life cycle costing a radical approach (CIRIA Report no 112).** Construction Research and Information Association, 1991.

Five steps to successful health and safety management. Health and Safety Executive, HSE Books 1992.

Framework for action: agenda for the estate. NHS in Scotland, Management Executive, Scottish Office 1994.

Greengard, S. **Making a virtual office reality.** Personnel Journal, 1994, Sept, p66-74.

Hammer, M. and Champney, J. **Re-engineering the corporation.** Brealey Publishing, 1993.

Hospital accreditation programme organisational standards and criteria. King's Fund Organisational Audit, 1994.

Huws, U. **Teleworking in Britain: a report to the employment department.** Employment Department, 1993.

Lathrop, P.J. **Restructuring healthcare: the patient focused paradigm.** Jossey-Bass, 1993.

NHS: A service with ambitions. Department of Health, The Stationery Office, 1996.

The Performance and cost managed building: Final Report, LINK/CMR Research Project no 4. Centre for Facilities Management, November 1993.

Quinn, R.E. **Beyond rational management.** Jossey-Bass, 1988.

Relating FM to organisational performance. Associate Company Research Report, Centre for Facilities Management, September 1995.

Schlezinger, L.A. and Hasket. **The service driven company.** Harvard Business Review, 1991, Sept/Oct.

Stevens, Katrina. **FM solutions for the millenium.** Facilities management casebook '96, Blenheim Business Publications, 1995.

Thinking about facilities management. Centre for Facilities Management, Business Round Table 1996.

Thomson, R. **Managing people.** Institute of Management, Butterworth-Heinemann Ltd., 1993.

Whitfield, M. **Telework trend gains momentum.** The Independent, 1993, Home News, p2.

Woodcock, M. **Team development manual.** Gower, 1993.

Working for patients. Department of Health, The Stationery Office 1989.

Other publications in this series

01 – Design for patient-focused care, Nov 93.

02 – Buildings for the day care of older people, Feb 94.

03 – Effective heat and power strategies for healthcare premises, Apr 94.

04 – NHS use of commercial premises, Mar 94.

05 – Design against crime: a strategic approach to hospital planning, Jun 94.

06 – Operational commissioning strategy – a manager's guide, Dec 95.

07 – Day surgery case study, Apr 95.

08 – Minimal access therapy, Feb 96.

09 – Fire safety – cost or benefit?, Feb 95.

10 – Rapid construction, Mar 96.

11 – Environmental management in healthcare, Feb 95.

12 – Acute care at home: estate implications, Mar 96.

13 – Ambulatory care and diagnostic centres: the experience of Central Middlesex Hospital, Jun 96.

14 – Disability access, Jul 96.

16 – Re-engineering the facilities management service, Mar 96.

19 – A design guide for residential care and nursing homes, in preparation.

20 – Access audits of primary healthcare facilities, Mar 97.

21 – Car parking, Sep 96.

26 – Refurbishment for natural ventilation, Mar 98.

27 – Reducing energy consumption in oversized plant, Mar 98.

29 – Materials management (supply, storage and distribution) in healthcare facilities, Mar 98.

About NHS Estates

NHS Estates is an Executive Agency of the Department of Health and is involved with all aspects of health estate management, development and maintenance. The Agency has a dynamic fund of knowledge which it has acquired during 35 years of working in the field. Using this knowledge NHS Estates has developed products which are unique in range and depth. These are described below. NHS Estates also makes its experience available to the field through its consultancy services.

Enquiries about NHS Estates should be addressed to:
NHS Estates, Publications Unit, Department of Health,
1 Trevelyan Square, Boar Lane, Leeds LS1 6AE.
Telephone 0113 254 7000.
http://www.open.govt.uk/nhest/hpage.htm

Some NHS Estates products

Activity DataBase – a computerised briefing and design system for use in health buildings, applicable to both new build and refurbishment schemes. *NHS Estates*

Design Guides – complementary to Health Building Notes, Design Guides provide advice for planners and designers about subjects not appropriate to the Health Building Notes series. *SO*

Estatecode – user manual for managing a health estate. Includes a recommended methodology for property appraisal and provides a basis for integration of the estate into corporate business planning. *SO*

Concode – outlines proven methods of selecting contracts and commissioning consultants. Reflects official policy on contract procedures. *SO*

Health Building Notes – advice for project teams procuring new buildings and adapting or extending existing buildings. *SO*

Health Guidance Notes – an occasional series of publications which respond to changes in Department of Health policy or reflect changing NHS operational management. Each deals with a specific topic and is complementary to a related HTM. *SO*

Health Technical Memoranda – guidance on the design, installation and running of specialised building service systems, and on specialised building components. *SO*

Health Facilities Notes – debate current and topical issues of concern across all areas of healthcare provision. *SO*

Encode – shows how to plan and implement a policy of energy efficiency in a building. *SO*

Firecode – for policy, technical guidance and specialist aspects of fire precautions. *SO*

Capital Investment Manual Database – software support for managing the capital programme. Compatible with Capital Investment Manual. *NHS Estates*

Model Engineering Specifications – comprehensive advice used in briefing consultants, contractors and suppliers of healthcare engineering services to meet Departmental policy and best practice guidance. *NHS Estates*

Quarterly Briefing – gives a regular overview on the construction industry and an outlook on how this may affect building projects in the health sector, in particular the impact on business prices. Also provides information on new and revised cost allowances for health buildings. Published four times a year; available on subscription direct from NHS Estates. *NHS Estates*

Items noted "SO" can be purchased from The Stationery Office Bookshops in London (post orders to PO Box 276, SW8 5DT), Edinburgh, Belfast, Cardiff, Manchester, Birmingham and Bristol or through good booksellers.

NHS Estates consultancy service

Designed to meet a range of needs from advice on the oversight of estates management functions to a much fuller collaboration for particularly innovative or exemplary projects.

Enquiries should be addressed to: NHS Estates Consultancy Service (address as above).

Printed in the United Kingdom for The Stationery Office
J41833 3/98 C6 9385 7738

NHS Estates

An Executive Agency of the Department of Health

Department of Health
1 Trevelyan Square
Boar Lane
Leeds
LS1 6AE
Fax 0113 254 7299
Telephone 0113 254 7000

Dear Customer

ꟷLD

At NHS Estates, we constantly strive to produce publications that are relevant to the demands of the NHS and our worldwide healthcare customers.

It would help us to provide you with a better service if you could set aside a few minutes to complete the questionnaire on the reverse, fold as shown and return in a window envelope.

Thank you for your comments.

Kate Priestley
Chief Executive

ꟷLD

KATE PRIESTLEY
CHIEF EXECUTIVE
NHS ESTATES
FREEPOST LS 5588
LEEDS
LS1 1YY

March 1998 – HFN 17: A business approach to facilities management

Publication title .... Date ....

Reader details

Name ....

Position ....

Organisation ....

Address ....

.... Postcode ....

Telephone ....

Please tick the appropriate box	Very Good	Good	Fair	Poor
Appropriateness of subject	❑	❑	❑	❑
Met my need	❑	❑	❑	❑
Clarity of presentation	❑	❑	❑	❑
Quality of content	❑	❑	❑	❑
Value for money	❑	❑	❑	❑
Overall rating of the publication	❑	❑	❑	❑

Will you be purchasing future editions in the series? YES ❑ NO ❑

Other comments/areas for improvement?

....

....

Do you have any suggested subjects for the future?

....

....

Do you receive copies of our quarterly Newslink newsletter? YES ❑ NO ❑

Do you wish to receive a copy? YES ❑ NO ❑

Have you purchased other products/services from us recently?

Please tick

Other publications	❑	**Activity DataBase**	❑
Consultancy services	❑	**Wims software enhancements**	❑
Other software products	❑	**Other: please specify**	❑

Are there other ways in which NHS Estates can assist you?

....

....

....

How did you receive your copy of this document?

Sent/issued by NHSE ❑ **Purchased from SO** ❑